Mechanisms for Organizational Behavior Change to Address the Needs of People Living with Alzheimer's Disease and Related Dementias

Crystal J. Bell, Austen Applegate,
Lyle Carrera, Tracy Lustig, and Carol
Berkower, *Rapporteurs*

Board on Health Care Services

Health and Medicine Division

Proceedings of a Workshop

NATIONAL ACADEMIES PRESS 500 Fifth Street, NW, Washington, DC 20001

This activity was supported by contracts between the National Academy of Sciences and the National Institutes of Health (contract no. HHSN263201800029I, task order no. 75N98021F00010). Any opinions, findings, conclusions, or recommendations expressed in this publication do not necessarily reflect the views of any organization or agency that provided support for the project.

International Standard Book Number-13: 978-0-309-69569-5
International Standard Book Number-10: 0-309-69569-4
Digital Object Identifier: https://doi.org/10.17226/26772

This publication is available from the National Academies Press, 500 Fifth Street, NW, Keck 360, Washington, DC 20001; (800) 624-6242 or (202) 334-3313; http://www.nap.edu.

Copyright 2022 by the National Academy of Sciences. National Academies of Sciences, Engineering, and Medicine and National Academies Press and the graphical logos for each are all trademarks of the National Academy of Sciences. All rights reserved.

Printed in the United States of America.

Suggested citation: National Academies of Sciences, Engineering, and Medicine. 2022. *Mechanisms for organizational behavior change to address the needs of people living with Alzheimer's disease and related dementias: Proceedings of a workshop.* Washington, DC: The National Academies Press. https://doi.org/10.17226/26772.

The **National Academy of Sciences** was established in 1863 by an Act of Congress, signed by President Lincoln, as a private, nongovernmental institution to advise the nation on issues related to science and technology. Members are elected by their peers for outstanding contributions to research. Dr. Marcia McNutt is president.

The **National Academy of Engineering** was established in 1964 under the charter of the National Academy of Sciences to bring the practices of engineering to advising the nation. Members are elected by their peers for extraordinary contributions to engineering. Dr. John L. Anderson is president.

The **National Academy of Medicine** (formerly the Institute of Medicine) was established in 1970 under the charter of the National Academy of Sciences to advise the nation on medical and health issues. Members are elected by their peers for distinguished contributions to medicine and health. Dr. Victor J. Dzau is president.

The three Academies work together as the **National Academies of Sciences, Engineering, and Medicine** to provide independent, objective analysis and advice to the nation and conduct other activities to solve complex problems and inform public policy decisions. The National Academies also encourage education and research, recognize outstanding contributions to knowledge, and increase public understanding in matters of science, engineering, and medicine.

Learn more about the National Academies of Sciences, Engineering, and Medicine at **www.nationalacademies.org**.

Consensus Study Reports published by the National Academies of Sciences, Engineering, and Medicine document the evidence-based consensus on the study's statement of task by an authoring committee of experts. Reports typically include findings, conclusions, and recommendations based on information gathered by the committee and the committee's deliberations. Each report has been subjected to a rigorous and independent peer-review process, and it represents the position of the National Academies on the statement of task.

Proceedings published by the National Academies of Sciences, Engineering, and Medicine chronicle the presentations and discussions at a workshop, symposium, or other event convened by the National Academies. The statements and opinions contained in proceedings are those of the participants and are not endorsed by other participants, the planning committee, or the National Academies.

Rapid Expert Consultations published by the National Academies of Sciences, Engineering, and Medicine are authored by subject-matter experts on narrowly focused topics that can be supported by a body of evidence. The discussions contained in rapid expert consultations are considered those of the authors and do not contain policy recommendations. Rapid expert consultations are reviewed by the institution before release.

For information about other products and activities of the National Academies, please visit www.nationalacademies.org/about/whatwedo.

PLANNING COMMITTEE FOR A WORKSHOP ON MECHANISMS FOR ORGANIZATIONAL BEHAVIOR CHANGE TO ADDRESS THE NEEDS OF PEOPLE LIVING WITH ALZHEIMER'S DISEASE AND RELATED DEMENTIAS[1]

RICHARD G. FRANK (*Chair*), Senior Fellow, Economic Studies, Brookings Institution; Director, USC-Brookings Schaeffer Initiative on Health Policy; and Margaret T. Morris Professor of Health Economics, Emeritus, Harvard Medical School
ELISABETH BELMONT, Corporate Counsel, MaineHealth
TERRY FULMER, President, John A. Hartford Foundation
SCOTT HALPERN, John M. Eisenberg Professor of Medicine, Epidemiology, and Medical Ethics and Health Policy, University of Pennsylvania
SHARON K. INOUYE, Director, Aging Brain Center, Hinda and Arthur Marcus Institute for Aging Research, Hebrew SeniorLife; Milton and Shirley F. Levy Family Chair and Professor of Medicine, Harvard Medical School
FAITH MITCHELL, Institute Fellow, Urban Institute
JULIE ROBISON, Professor of Medicine, Center on Aging, University of Connecticut School of Medicine

Project Staff

CRYSTAL BELL, Associate Program Officer
AUSTEN APPLEGATE, Research Associate (from May 2022)
LORI BRENIG, Research Associate (June 2022–July 2022)
TORRIE BROWN, Senior Program Assistant (June 2022–July 2022)
LYLE CARRERA, Research Associate (from June 2022)
MOLLY CHECKSFIELD DORRIES, Program Officer
TRACY LUSTIG, Senior Program Officer
RUKSHANA GUPTA, Senior Program Assistant (March 2022–June 2022)
ARZOO TAYYEB, Finance Business Partner
SHARYL NASS, Senior Board Director

Consultant

CAROL BERKOWER, Consulting Writer

---

[1] The National Academies of Sciences, Engineering, and Medicine's planning committees are solely responsible for organizing the workshop, identifying topics, and choosing speakers. The responsibility for the published Proceedings of a Workshop rests with the workshop rapporteurs and the institution.

BOARD ON HEALTH CARE SERVICES[1]

DONALD M. BERWICK (*Chair*), Harvard Medical School
ANDREW B. BINDMAN, Kaiser Foundation Health Plan, Inc., and Hospitals
NIRANJAN BOSE, Gates Ventures
NEIL S. CALMAN, Institute for Family Health and Icahn School of Medicine at Mount Sinai
PAUL CHUNG, Kaiser Permanente Bernard J. Tyson School of Medicine
PATRICIA M. DAVIDSON, University of Wollongong
MARTHA DAVIGLUS, University of Illinois at Chicago
JENNIFER E. DEVOE, Oregon Health & Science University
RICHARD G. FRANK, Harvard Medical School and University of Southern California–Brookings Schaeffer Initiative on Health Policy
CINDY GILLESPIE, Arkansas Department of Human Services
ELMER E. HUERTA, The George Washington University Cancer Center
LAUREN HUGHES, Farley Health Center and University of Colorado
SHARON K. INOUYE, Harvard Medical School and Hebrew SeniorLife
JOHN R. LUMPKIN, Blue Cross and Blue Shield of North Carolina Foundation
FAITH MITCHELL, Urban Institute
DAVID B. PRYOR, Ascension Clinical Holdings (retired)
JULIE ROBISON, University of Connecticut School of Medicine
WILLIAM M. SAGE, University of Texas at Austin
HARDEEP SINGH, Michael E. DeBakey VA Medical Center and Baylor College of Medicine
LAURIE ZEPHRYIN, The Commonwealth Fund
MICHAEL ZUBKOFF, Dartmouth College

---

[1] The National Academies of Sciences, Engineering, and Medicine's forums and roundtables do not issue, review, or approve individual documents. The responsibility for the published Proceedings of a Workshop rests with the workshop rapporteurs and the institution.

Reviewers

This Proceedings of a Workshop was reviewed in draft form by individuals chosen for their diverse perspectives and technical expertise. The purpose of this independent review is to provide candid and critical comments that will assist the National Academies of Sciences, Engineering, and Medicine in making each published proceedings as sound as possible and to ensure that it meets the institutional standards for quality, objectivity, evidence, and responsiveness to the charge. The review comments and draft manuscript remain confidential to protect the integrity of the process.

We thank the following individuals for their review of this proceedings:

SARAH DULANEY, University of California, San Francisco
GARY P. EPSTEIN-LUBOW, Brown University

Although the reviewers listed above provided many constructive comments and suggestions, they were not asked to endorse the content of the proceedings nor did they see the final draft before its release. The review of this proceedings was overseen by **LINDA A. MCCAULEY,** Emory University. She was responsible for making certain that an independent examination of this proceedings was carried out in accordance with standards of the National Academies and that all review comments were carefully considered. Responsibility for the final content rests entirely with the rapporteurs and the National Academies.

We also thank staff member Connie Citro for reading and providing helpful comments on this manuscript.

Acknowledgments

The National Academies of Sciences, Engineering, and Medicine's Board on Health Care Services wishes to express its sincere gratitude to the planning committee chair Lauren S. Hughes for her valuable contributions to the development and organization of this workshop. The board wishes to thank all the members of the planning committee, who collaborated to ensure a workshop complete with informative presentations and rich discussions. Finally, the board wishes to thank the speakers and moderators, who generously shared their expertise and their time with workshop participants. Funding from the National Institutes of Health made this workshop possible.

Contents

1	INTRODUCTION	1
2	KEYNOTE PRESENTATIONS	7
3	DEFINING QUALITY	19
4	TRANSFORMING THE ROLE OF PAYMENT SYSTEM INCENTIVES TO IMPROVE QUALITY	33
5	EVIDENCE ON THE EFFECT OF EXISTING MODELS AND RESEARCH AND INNOVATION TO ADDRESS GAPS IN DATA AND EVIDENCE	47
6	CREATING CHANGE	61
7	FINAL THOUGHTS	73

APPENDIXES
A References   79
B Statement of Task   87
C Workshop Agenda   89
D Biographical Sketches of the Speakers and Committee Members   93
E Acronyms and Abbreviations   107

1

Introduction[1]

The Alzheimer's Association estimates that 6.5 million Americans age 65 and older (10.7 percent) have Alzheimer's disease in 2022, with related dementias affecting an additional 2 to 3 million individuals. Prevalence is projected to double by 2060 (Alzheimer's Association, 2022). Patients diagnosed with Alzheimer's disease and related dementias (ADRD) rely on family members, their community, and the health care system for progressively increasing support over the course of their disease. These people receive care through a frequently siloed health care system across hospitals, nursing homes, ambulatory care settings, and long-term care settings, as well as community- and home-based care. As the number of people living with a diagnosis of ADRD continues to grow, so does the need to provide better support for these people and their caregivers.

Evidence-based, high-quality care can enhance the quality of life for both individuals living with ADRD and their caregivers. It also can decrease the likelihood of adverse events, such as falls, hospital-acquired infections, and hospital-induced delirium that have the potential to exacerbate disease progression. The advent of payment policies, such as accountable care organiza-

---

[1] The planning committee's role was limited to planning the workshop, and the Proceedings of a Workshop has been prepared by the workshop rapporteurs as a factual summary of what occurred at the workshop. Statements, recommendations, and opinions expressed are those of individual presenters and participants, and are not necessarily endorsed or verified by the National Academies of Sciences, Engineering, and Medicine, and they should not be construed as reflecting any group consensus.

tions (ACOs) have led to hospitals and health care systems having a financial interest in promoting quality care for people living with ADRD.

The National Institute on Aging (NIA) Division of Behavioral and Social Research suggests that organizational behavior change will be needed for health care systems to integrate all of the services and supports required to provide high-quality care for people with ADRD. NIA believes payment policy is one of the policy tools that could facilitate the necessary organizational behavior change to improve quality of care for people with ADRD. However, there remains a gap in knowledge about how to effectively use financial incentives to change hospital and health care system organizational behavior in a way that is responsive to the needs of people living with ADRD.

NIA sponsored a workshop hosted by the National Academies of Sciences, Engineering, and Medicine to explore mechanisms to improve the quality of care for people living with ADRD and the potential of innovative payment models to incentivize health care systems to make the necessary systemic changes.[2] National Academies of Sciences, Engineering, and Medicine project staff from the Board on Health Care Services (HCS) and the Board on Behavioral, Cognitive, and Sensory Sciences (BBCSS) assembled a preliminary working group that consisted of experts in the pertinent fields of study to determine the scope of the workshop and identify key topics to be addressed at the workshop. A separate planning committee that included several members of the preliminary working group developed the agenda for workshop sessions, selected and invited speakers, moderated panel discussions, and gave presentations. The hybrid workshop was held concurrently at the National Academy of Sciences Building in Washington, D.C., and online on May 23–24, 2022. The workshop convened a diverse array of experts in fields including nursing, geriatrics, health care economics, health care services research, quality measurement, social work, medical ethics, law, health care finance, and health care policy. Participants came from a variety of settings, including academic research institutions, government agencies, nonpartisan research foundations, and medical care centers. The workshop was open to the public. The recorded webcast has been archived online.[3]

---

[2] See https://www.nationalacademies.org/our-work/mechanisms-for-organizational-behavior-change-to-address-the-needs-of-people-living-with-alzheimers-disease-and-related-dementias-a-workshop (accessed September 28, 2022).

[3] See https://www.nationalacademies.org/event/05-23-2022/mechanisms-for-organizational-behavior-change-to-address-the-needs-of-people-living-with-alzheimers-disease-and-related-dementias-a-workshop#sectionWebFriendly (accessed September 28, 2022).

ORGANIZATION OF THE PROCEEDINGS

This workshop proceedings was developed by rapporteurs based on recordings, transcripts, and slides from the workshop. It represents a high-level summary of the presentations and discussions. This proceedings document is divided into seven chapters that reflect the keynote presentations, each of the four workshop sessions, and the final panel discussion, which included closing reflections. Box 1 is the rapporteurs' list of summarized points made by individual identified speakers. The list of references is in Appendix A, the workshop statement of task is in Appendix B, and the workshop agenda is in Appendix C. The biographies of workshop planning committee members and invited speakers can be found in Appendix D, and a list of acronyms and abbreviations can be found in Appendix E.

BOX 1
Key Considerations Highlighted by Individual Workshop Participants for Improved Quality of Care and Support for People Living With Alzheimer's Disease and Related Dementias and Their Caregivers

Financial mechanisms
- Current payment models do not reflect the roles that frontline Alzheimer's disease and related dementias (ADRD) caregivers and community-based partners play in providing effective, person-centered care for people living with ADRD (Ferrell, Reuben, Robison, Vladeck).
- Financial incentives can be used to encourage use of evidence-based models of comprehensive ADRD care (Reuben, Robison, Vladeck).
- People living with ADRD and their caregivers across the income and resource continuum may be better supported via public funding for long-term care (Inouye, McEvoy), as well as by improved interagency coordination, such as between the Centers for Medicare and Medicaid Services (CMS) and the Administration for Community Living (ACL) (McEvoy).
- Payment and policy changes can help support and develop the ADRD care workforce (Lamont, Vladeck).
- The current ADRD care system often does not adequately involve or support informal caregivers, though caregivers provide important support for care transitions, mental health and well-being, and episodic care (Frank, Gwyther, Inouye, Largent, Lenz Lock, McEvoy).

continued

BOX 1 Continued

Research for future financial mechanisms
- Additional research would be beneficial to gain insight into to how various payment models, delivery systems, and regulatory reforms interact to affect care for people living with ADRD across the care continuum (Hollmann, Lenz Lock, Navathe, Sherry).
- New payment models designed to improve the quality of care and support for people living with ADRD and their caregivers may be best tested through smaller pilot studies due to the unique and complicated nature of providing such care (Navathe).
- Specific areas of interest for future research include Medicare payment streams (Lenz Lock), episodic care (Navathe), assisted living facilities (Sherry), and caregiver support (Navathe).
- The existing evidence base for improving quality of care through new financial mechanisms and care models could be investigated for key components that could be integrated into an ADRD specific model (Fulmer, McEvoy).

Data collection
- Tools to measure quality of care throughout the care continuum can help set standards and support value-based payment models (Lamont, Schneider).
- Outcomes regarding patients' goals and expectations could offer valuable insight that can supplement clinical outcome data (Ferrell, Hollmann, Lenz Lock, Pelton, Robison, Schneider, Sherry).
- Community involvement can help develop better quality measures for health equity accreditation programs (Schneider).
- Data infrastructures and analysis systems in use by other industries may be applicable to improving the quality of care for people living with ADRD (Hansen, Hollmann, Lamont, Schneider, Robison).

Implementation and scaling up
- Regulatory obstacles can hinder uptake of evidence-based programs, and strategies to overcome these obstacles might encourage broader implementation (Epstein-Lubow, Inouye).
- Pragmatic trials of home care options can offer insights into improving flexibility in the ADRD care system (Inouye).
- Scaling up models may require an institutionally based strategy at the state and regional levels (McEvoy, Vladek).
- International examples can provide insights into what "good" ADRD care looks like, such as multidisciplinary and collaborative approaches that involve both paid and unpaid caregivers (Jang, Robison).
- Existing tools, such as those from AARP and USAging, can help encourage the dissemination of promising practices (Lenz Lock).

BOX 1 Continued

- Partnerships between health care providers and community-based organizations can support implementation of new care models and tailor them to diverse populations (Pelton).

The Dementia care workforce
- The National Academies of Sciences, Engineering, and Medicine nursing home consensus study (2022) suggests changes to the nursing home workforce that could improve quality of care for people with ADRD (Ferrell, Vladek).
- Training and professional development for staff of nursing homes and other long-term care facilities could help address the ADRD care workforce shortage (Ferrell, Fullmer, Hollmann).
- Team-based models of care for people with ADRD could benefit from including family caregivers, community-based caregivers, health care professionals, long-term care providers, and other professions (Gwyther, Hollmann, Lamont, Schneider).
- ADRD care would be useful to include in training curricula for physicians and other health care staff (Lamont, Reuben, Vladek).

Inequities in dementia care
- Targeted research funding and education are possible tools to reduce inequities experienced by people living with ADRD and their caregivers (Mitchell, Robison).
- Focusing on the identities of people with ADRD when designing care and program evaluation can support equity (Pelton, Seshamani).
- People living with ADRD that are without caregivers, friends, or family to support them are particularly vulnerable to inequities (Largent, Seshamani).
- Culturally sensitive care is an important part of health care professional training that could support improved quality of care for people with ADRD (Ferrell, Mitchell).

Note: This list is the rapporteurs' summary of points made by the individual speakers identified, and the statements have not been endorsed or verified by the National Academies of Sciences, Engineering, and Medicine. They are not intended to reflect a consensus among workshop participants.

[a] Speakers used a variety of terms throughout the workshop to refer to the people who provide support to someone living with Alzheimer's disease and related dementias and have a personal relationship with that person instead of an employment-based relationship. Examples include family caregiver, informal caregiver, caregiver, or unpaid caregiver. This reflects the diversity of family caregivers. Generally, this proceedings uses the term that was used by the respective speaker. In cases where speakers referred specifically to paid caregivers, that is indicated in the text.

BACKGROUND

Richard Frank, director of the University of Southern California-Brookings Schaeffer Initiative on Health Policy, offered a brief description of the central goal of the workshop as described in the statement of task. The workshop seeks to gain insight from various experts to develop an understanding of how various tools could be applied to facilitate improvements in care delivery and support for people living with ADRD as well as their caregivers and families.

Melinda Kelley, acting deputy director of NIA, and Theresa Kim, social and behavioral science program official at NIA, offered opening remarks that described the relevance of this workshop to NIA. Kelley noted that the breadth of topics that will be discussed during the workshop, such as evidence regarding defining quality care for people living with ADRD; identification of gaps in data for payment models; and the application of social sciences toward developing payment models that promote high-quality care will provide NIA with valuable insight as it considers future research priorities. Kim explained that the Division of Behavioral and Social Research (BSR), an extramural division of NIA, supports social, behavioral, and economic research on the processes of aging at individual and societal levels. BSR receives input from experts, including the National Advisory Council on Aging (NACA), which recommends future directions every 5 years. This workshop is relevant to several of NACA's 2019 recommendations, including supporting research on individual and organizational change and research on improving care for patients with ADRD and their caregivers. Kim noted that while many health care, public health, and social service systems are redesigning their programs and processes to address the current siloed nature of care and service delivery, there remains a gap in understanding how to reliably implement organizational change initiatives to better serve people living with ADRD. She explained that NIA hopes to use what is learned at this workshop to guide the development of research into policy options to incentivize improved care and support for people with ADRD and their caregivers.

2

Keynote Presentations

DEMENTIA CARE: GETTING IT RIGHT FOR EVERYONE

David Reuben, director of the University of California-Los Angeles (UCLA) Alzheimer's disease and dementia care program and director of UCLA's Multi-campus Program in Geriatric Medicine and Gerontology, offered an overview of dementia and dementia care in the United States. He began by explaining that *dementia* is an umbrella term for loss of memory and other thinking abilities that reaches a level of severity sufficient to interfere with daily life. Alzheimer's disease (AD) is responsible for 60 to 80 percent of all dementias, with the remaining cases attributable to Lewy body dementia, vascular dementia, frontotemporal dementia, or other neurological disorders, such as Parkinson's and Huntington's diseases. Multiple disorders may coexist in the same individual, producing mixed dementia. AD affects 5 percent of individuals age 65 to 74, 13 percent of those age 75 to 84, and 33 percent of those age 85 and older (Alzheimer's Association, 2022). The number of people diagnosed with AD is expected to reach 7.2 million by 2025 (Alzheimer's Association, 2022). Reuben noted that rates of AD diagnosis are higher in people who identify as Black or Latinx than in those that identify as White or not Latinx (Alzheimer's Association, 2022).

Reuben explained that in 2011, the National Institute on Aging (NIA) and the Alzheimer's Association redefined AD to recognize three distinct stages of disease, which may be distinguished by biomarkers (Alzheimer's Association, 2022). The first stage is referred to as the preclinical stage, progression from which is defined by changes in certain biomarkers (as compared to individuals with normal cognition). The second stage is referred to as mild cognitive impairment (MCI) and is characterized by impairment in cognition mild enough to preserve overall function, and biomarkers of AD may be present. The third stage, dementia, is characterized by impairments in both cognition and function, and biomarkers may help to exclude AD as the cause of cognitive and functional impairment. In 2017, 46.7 million Americans were estimated to have positive biomarkers for one of these stages (McDade et al., 2020). The vast majority of these were in the preclinical or MCI stage (Brookmeyer et al., 2018). However, 10 to 15 percent of people with MCI convert to dementia each year, and roughly 50 percent convert in 5 years (Alzheimer's Association, 2022). He emphasized that this represents a rapid progression of disease severity and prevalence.

Reuben explained that the natural history of AD is characterized by progressive cognitive decline, as measured by the Mini Mental State Examination, at a rate of approximately 10 percent per year (Pangman et al., 2000). Approximately 30 to 50 percent of people with Alzheimer's disease and related dementias (ADRD) experience non-cognitive symptoms (Masters et al., 2015). Those symptoms, including apathy, depression, agitation or aggression, sleep disorders, and delusions, can be very disruptive and last for years. Survival after the onset of symptoms is 3 to 12 years (Larson et al., 2004; Ryman et al., 2014). The currently available tests for predicting AD are of reasonable quality and continue to improve, said Reuben. As methods of detecting dementia improve, so are strategies for managing the disease. Reuben expects the current modalities of detection, treatment, and support will be supplemented with risk factor identification, monitoring, and prevention by 2030. He compared the use of biomarkers to detect those at risk for AD to that of serum cholesterol and other blood biomarkers in the management of coronary artery disease as a model for disease prediction.

Reuben next highlighted the cost of ADRD care in relation to quality of care. Total annual payments for ADRD care are $321 billion as of 2022, of which $206 billion has been paid by Medicare and Medicaid (Alzheimer's Association, 2022). Patients and families contribute about a quarter of that payment total ($81 billion) in the form of out-of-pocket payments (Alzheimer's Association, 2022). People living with ADRD also receive a great deal of care that is not paid for by any entity. In 2021, unpaid caregivers provided approximately 16 billion hours of care, valued at $271.6 billion (Alzheimer's Association, 2022). The average lifetime cost of care for a person living with ADRD is $371,621 (Alzheimer's Association, 2022). He noted that despite its high cost, there is substantial opportunity for improvement in the quality of paid ADRD care, citing a published analysis that employed the Assessing Care of Vulnerable Elders (ACOVE-3) and Physician Consortium for Performance Improvement (PCPI) quality indicators (American Medical Association, 2011; Jennings et al., 2016; Wenger et al., 2007). This analysis graded the quality of dementia care provided by community-based physicians at 38 percent; addition of a nurse practitioner increased quality to 60 percent (Reuben et al., 2019). However, adding a nurse practitioner or physician's assistant who focused solely on dementia increased the quality of care grade to 92 percent (Jennings et al., 2016).

Reuben emphasized that dementia is a lifetime disease with no cure, which requires caregivers to adapt to the changing nature of their role, particularly related to decision making, as the disease progresses. During early disease, while the person living with dementia still has cognitive capacity to do so, they should be included in advance-care planning and other decision making, such as participation in clinical trials. He added that care goals during early disease should focus on maintaining the highest level of independence that is feasible for all involved (including the family and caregivers); treating the disease; managing potentially contentious issues, such as driving; managing symptoms; and managing comorbidities. In the later stages of disease, as cognition declines, families and caregivers must become responsible for making progressively more, and eventually all decisions.

Reuben explained that a caregiver is the most important person in the life of an individual with dementia. However, he said over 50 percent of caregivers develop depression. Several caregiver training and support programs have been found to reduce caregiver depression and increase the quality of care, such as Resources for Enhancing Alzheimer's Caregiver Health II (REACH II);[1] the New York University (NYU) Caregiver Intervention;[2] and programs run by the Alzheimer's Association (Belle et al., 2006; Gaugler et al., 2018).[3] These programs have been found to enhance caregiver knowledge, well-being, and confidence; increase the duration of time from diagnosis to institutionalization; and reduce behavioral symptoms of people living with ADRD. However, Reuben also noted that there is a financial cost for these programs. They are not well integrated into health care systems, and further pragmatic testing is needed. He suggested that the additional pragmatic testing could be a good opportunity for collaboration with the NIA Impact Collaboratory.[4]

Reuben highlighted several new models of comprehensive ADRD care. Many of these models focus on the patient–caregiver dyad and are either community based, such as the Benjamin Rose Institute Care Consultation

---

[1] See https://www.apa.org/pi/about/publications/caregivers/practice-settings/intervention/reach-protocol (accessed August 30, 2022).

[2] See https://www.caregiver.org/resource/new-york-university-caregivers-program/ (accessed August 30, 2022).

[3] See https://www.alz.org/help-support/caregiving (accessed July 5, 2022).

[4] See https://impactcollaboratory.org (accessed July 5, 2022).

(BRICC),[5] Johns Hopkins Maximizing Independence (MIND) at Home,[6] and the University of California-San Francisco (UCSF) Care Ecosystem.[7] Others are based in the health system, such as the Indiana University Healthy Aging Brain Center (HABC),[8] the UCLA Alzheimer's and Dementia Care Program (ADC),[9] and Emory University's Integrated Memory Care Clinic (IMCC)[10] (Clevenger et al., 2018; French et al., 2014; Reuben et al., 2019). While each of these models differs in certain respects (see Table 2-1), they all employ what Reuben described as the essential pillars of comprehensive ADRD care:

- Continuous monitoring and assessment
- Ongoing care plans
- Psychosocial interventions for both people living with ADRD and caregivers
- Self-management
- Treatment of related conditions
- Coordination of care

Most of the models have been shown to benefit both patients and caregivers, and while they cost money to administer, they also produce savings. Despite their effectiveness, these programs are not widely available. Reuben cited several possible barriers that may be responsible for limited adoption. One challenge is the misaligned incentives that can occur when initial costs associated with implementation are not well reimbursed, and cost savings associated with the models are instead realized by stakeholders that did not invest in the implementation process. Other reasons that he cited for limited adoption of these models include the need to train practitioners; the need to identify, vet, and establish a payment stream for community-based partners; and inertia.

Reuben offered an example of the interaction between severity of ADRD and cost of care based on 2017 data from 5,000 patients living with ADRD in UCLA's Population-Based Dementia Care Model. The model illustrates levels of dementia as a pyramid stratified by severity of disease (see Figure 2-1). The

---

[5] See https://benrose.org/-/bricareconsultation (accessed July 5, 2022).

[6] See http://www.mindathome.org (accessed July 5, 2022).

[7] See https://memory.ucsf.edu/research-trials/professional/care-ecosystem (accessed July 5, 2022).

[8] See https://www.eskenazihealth.edu/health-services/brain-center/aging-brain-care-program (accessed September 28, 2022).

[9] See https://www.uclahealth.org/dementia/ (accessed July 26 2022).

[10] See https://www.emoryhealthcare.org/centers-programs/integrated-memory-care-clinic/index.html (accessed September 28, 2022).

TABLE 2-1 Comparison of Select Dementia Care Models

	BRI CC	Care Ecosystem	MIND	HABC	UCLA ADC	IMCC
Structure/process						
Key personnel	SW, RN, MFT	Non-licensed APN, SW, pharmacist	Non-licensed RN, MD	Non-licensed MD, SW, RN, psychologist	NP, PA, MD	APN
Key personnel base	CBO	Community	Community	Health system	Health system	Health system
Face-to-face visits	No	No	Yes	Yes	Yes	Yes
Access 24/7/365	No	No	No	Yes	Yes	Yes
Communication with PCP	Mail, fax	Fax, phone	Phone, mail, fax	EHR, phone, mail	EHR, phone	N/A
Order writing	No	No	No	Yes	Yes	Yes
Benefits						
High quality of care	N/A	N/A	N/A	Yes	Yes	Yes
Patient benefit	Yes	Yes	Yes	Yes	Yes	NS
Caregiver benefit	Yes	Yes	Yes	Yes	Yes	NS
Costs of program	++	++	+++	+++	++++	++++
Cost savings, gross	++	++	None	++	++++	++++

NOTE: + = represent qualitative estimates, with a single + representing the least and four + representing the most; Non-licensed = personnel that are not licensed professionals, but usually have a bachelor's or master's degree in a nonclinical area; APN = advanced practice nurse; CBO = community-based organization; EHR = electronic health record; MD = medical doctor; MFT = marriage and family therapist; NP = nurse practitioner; PA = physician assistant; PCP = primary care provider; RN = registered nurse; SW = social worker.
SOURCE: Presented by David Reuben on May 23, 2022, at Mechanisms for Organizational Behavior Change to Address the Needs of People Living with Alzheimer's Disease and Related Dementias: A Workshop. Adapted from Lees Haggerty, K., G. Epstein-Lubow, L. H. Spragens, R. J. Stoeckle, L. C. Evertson, L. A. Jennings, and D. B. Reuben. 2020. Recommendations to improve payment policies for comprehensive dementia care. *Journal of the American Geriatrics Society* 68(11):2478-2485.

top of the pyramid represents the 1 percent of patients whose severe functional impairments, behavioral problems, and comorbidities require intensive individualized care that costs on average $186,000 annually. The cost of care for patients in the second tier averages $65,000 annually, while the cost of care for those in the third tier averages $20,000 annually. The patients in the second and third tier differ in their intensity of behavioral symptoms and hospital visits, but individuals in both tiers are likely to require a high- or low-intensity dementia care program, as well as neurological and psychiatric care. Patients in the fourth and fifth tiers typically have less intense behavioral symptoms and fewer hospital visits than those in the other three tiers and can rely on a less intensive and far less expensive dementia care program as well as caregiver education and monitoring. He noted that the fourth and fifth tiers of the pyramid may also represent an opportunity for incorporating referrals to community-based resources into patient care.

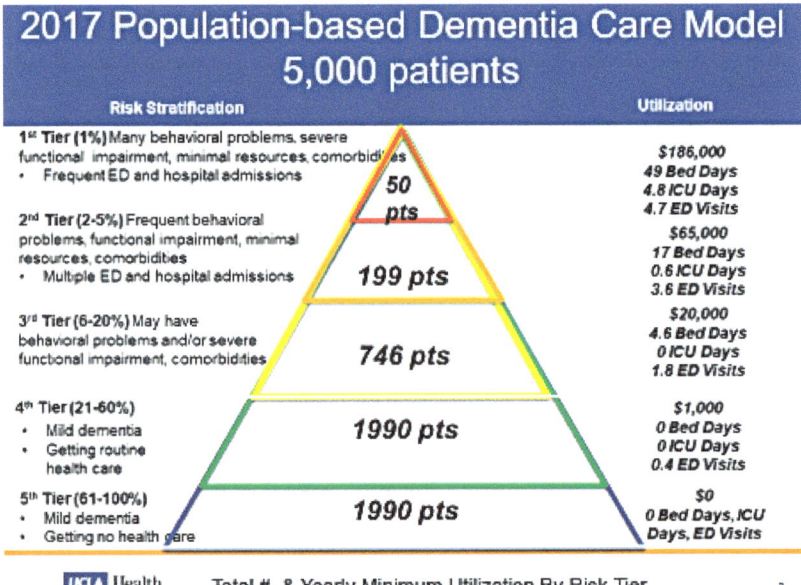

FIGURE 2-1 The pyramid of dementia care based on disease stratification and resource utilization
NOTE: ED = emergency department; pts = patients; ICU =intensive care unit.
SOURCE: Presented by David Reuben on May 23, 2022, at Mechanisms for Organizational Behavior Change to Address the Needs of People Living with Alzheimer's Disease and Related Dementias: A Workshop. Adapted from "How A Population-Based Approach Can Improve Dementia Care," *Health Affairs Blog*, May 8, 2019.

CONNECTING PAYMENT TO PRACTICE THROUGH MEDICARE

Meena Seshamani, director of the Center for Medicare at the Centers for Medicare and Medicaid Services, discussed its ongoing work and future opportunities to drive improvement in the quality of care for people with ADRD and support for their families and caregivers. She noted that Medicare has the power to propel systemic change due to the immense size of the program. Medicare covers 63 million people, including all Americans age 65 and older, as well as younger individuals with disabilities or end-stage renal disease. Medicare partners with more than one million clinicians and 6,000 hospitals and reimburses almost one trillion dollars in annual claims—about one in five health care dollars (CMS, 2022b). Approximately 11 percent of Medicare claims are for the care of people with ADRD (Hurd et al., 2013). She noted that these patients would benefit from a more holistic and less siloed approach to care.

Seshamani described Medicare's vision for better serving people with ADRD, their families, and caregivers as being organized into several categories. The first category is a recommitment to advancing health equity (Seshamani and Jacobs, 2022; Seshamani et al., 2022). People from groups that have been historically made vulnerable and are lacking in resources are frequently systemically overlooked. She opined that to address inequity at the level of the Center for Medicare's everyday operations it is essential that supporting those individuals remains central to operational decisions that affect system oversight, quality metrics, and navigability. The Center for Medicare is developing specific policies to address disparities in health care and to support health care organizations as they address those disparities. This includes designating 200 new physician residency slots in rural and underserved areas each year for the next five years (CMS, 2021).

The Center for Medicare is also seeking comment on a health equity index for Medicare Advantage insurance plans to ensure that those plans serve people from groups that have been historically made the most vulnerable (CMS, 2022a). Another category for Medicare's vision is focused on access to coverage and care, which has particular relevance to people with AD. Medicare has been able to use reimbursement to facilitate the integration of cognitive screening into covered beneficiaries' annual wellness visit. It is also seeking additional opportunities to use payments to encourage additional improvements in care, such as the integration of behavioral health care into primary care. She said the Center for Medicare is also considering strategies for using payments to achieve equity in behavioral health care and primary care, including addressing issues of language access and needs related to social determinants of health (social needs).

Seshamani explained that another category for Medicare's vision involves innovations to create more holistic models that facilitate higher quality care for more people. Accountable care organizations (ACOs) will play a central role in those efforts. She noted that ACOs emphasize a team-based holistic approach to care while attaining high quality metrics and generating shared cost savings. The Center for Medicare aims to bring all beneficiaries of traditional Medicare into an ACO by 2030. There will be a particular focus on increasing participation in ACOs in rural and underserved areas. However, she noted that improved quality of care for people with ADRD requires more than enrolling providers in these models. Therefore, the Center for Medicare is seeking to develop partnerships that will support those who care for people with ADRD. Opportunities to accomplish this include possible partnerships with the Health Resources and Services Administration (HRSA) and the Centers for Disease Control and Prevention (CDC) that could fund innovations on the community level that advance whole-person care for people with ADRD. She also noted that in order to increase momentum for system change, social services, health care, other support services, foundations and government grant makers, resources from ACO learning communities, and funding streams within CMS itself all need to be in alignment.

Seshamani emphasized the importance of research partnerships, noting the power of research tools to evaluate changes and reveal inequities that have emerged during the COVID-19 pandemic, such as the expansion of telehealth, the use of community health workers, and integration of public health into the traditional health care system. Research can identify areas where these changes were effective and what may need to be modified to make some changes more effective. Seshamani noted that researchers should evaluate every program change against the goals of advancing equity, furthering whole-person care, stewarding Medicare (reducing waste, fraud, and abuse), and preventing future complications. Finally, Seshamani encouraged an approach to care that extends beyond the medical office or hospital to include family, community, and social needs, in a manner that leads to better care, smarter spending, and improved health.

DISCUSSION

Addressing the Most Urgent Needs in ADRD Care

Richard Frank began the discussion by asking what evidence is needed to understand which policy levers are most crucial to facilitate systemic change to support improved quality of care for people with ADRD. Reuben responded that payment policy directed at improving quality of care should be comprehensive, instead of focusing on discrete services, and include nontraditional types of care to address the many services frequently needed by people with ADRD that are not covered by insurers. He noted that legislation has been introduced in the U.S. Congress related to the Center for Medicare and Medicaid Innovation (CMMI) studying alternative approaches for financing ADRD care. He added that care for people with ADRD requires a different approach than that applied to many other diseases, due to the inability of many patients to participate in their own decision making and the tremendous psychosocial and behavioral complications associated with ADRD. Seshamani added that several considerations should be evaluated prior to the large-scale implementation of new approaches, such as the movement of more care into the home setting that occurred during the COVID-19 pandemic. These considerations include identifying the target patient population, clarifying how the change will affect patient well-being, the patient's family members and other caregivers, patient-reported outcomes, health care outcomes, health care utilization, and health care spending.

Addressing Systemic Health Inequities

Jennie Chin Hansen asked how CMS could address the significant effect of ADRD on Black people that are dually eligible for Medicare and Medicaid, noting that people in this group have historically faced barriers to economic stability and health care inequities. Seshamani noted that Black people enrolled in Medicare have a higher rate of ADRD than other populations. She explained that addressing Medicare's daily operations with a focus on culture, language, and the environment in which a person is living while they are receiving care will help to address general issues of health inequity as well as the greater effects of ADRD on Black people. She noted that the CMS expansion of graduate medical education (GME) residencies in underserved areas reflects an effort to bring providers to settings where they are most needed. She added that CMS will gauge the effect of innovations on quality of care for Black enrollees in part through race and ethnicity data collected as part of Medicare Advantage and Medicare Part D enrollment.

Reuben noted health equity is a significant issue for caregivers and communities. People living with AD and their families frequently receive substantial support from their communities, which highlights the important role of ethnicity and culture, including local culture in ADRD care. He added that the important role of community support highlights the need for adequate reimbursement for the work done by community-based organizations. Bruce Vladeck, Greater New York Hospital Association and LiveOnNY, added that the workforce providing in-home care is disproportionately composed of people of color that identify as female. He said their compensation, training, and working conditions represent a significant equity issue. Reuben agreed, adding that many paid caregivers are immigrants, and many lack health care benefits or insurance in addition to other challenges related to their immigration status, creating an "extraordinarily complicated issue, but one that we need to tackle." Seshamani agreed on the importance of including caregivers in initiatives related to improving equity. She added that CMS, in cooperation with HRSA, has a role in efforts to support the health care workforce, including training and expanding the pipeline of future professional caregivers, and burnout prevention. She added that efforts should not overlook people she referred to as double caregivers, people that are employed as caregivers and also serve as caregivers at home.

Barriers to Innovation in Dementia Care

Sharon Inouye, Harvard Medical School and planning committee member, noted that effective models for ADRD care that reduce costs and improve quality of care exist and asked the speakers to address the major barriers to their implementation. Reuben began by explaining that he has spoken to 60 to 70 health care systems in his efforts to disseminate the UCLA Alzheimer's and Dementia Care Program.[11] He said that while many health care systems were generally supportive of the model and interested in its benefits, they were also concerned about the cost of the needed additional staff members, such as nurse practitioners. He described three common barriers to implementing these models. The first barrier, which he also mentioned in his presentation, is the initial cost of implementation, as the financial benefits of implementing these models are frequently accrued elsewhere in the health care system. The second barrier is the need to train practitioners, who are not often trained in this specific type of care. The third barrier is the need to provide adequate funding for community-based organizations to provide supports tailored to patients with ADRD and their families.

Seshamani, in response to the same question, explained the three types of authority that Medicare can engage to different degrees to facilitate adoption of these models (CMS, 2022c; Jaeger-Fine, 2020). The first is statutory authority. The Medicare program derives its authority via statute; some improvements require changes in the statute, which usually involve congressional action. The second is regulatory authority, as current statute gives Medicare regulatory authority. The third authority is direct effect on the provision of care by including support for training providers and caregivers, support for

---

[11] See https://www.uclahealth.org/dementia/ (accessed July 26, 2022).

local community partnerships, and increased engagement with family caregivers, said Seshamani.

Funding Care at Home

Peter Hollmann, Brown University and Lifespan Health Alliance, asked if funding programs designed for people with developmental disabilities might offer useful lessons for funding at-home care for people living with ADRD, particularly whether an approach similar to the Katie Beckett Medicaid Waiver or merging Medicare and Medicaid could be possible solutions. Hollmann opined that one of the greatest challenges related to providing people with ADRD care at home is paying for care provided by community-based organizations and paying for the long-term support services that are generally considered the obligation of the patient and their family but are often prohibitively expensive. Seshamani said that the Medicare and Medicaid coordination office is considering opportunities to improve care for dually eligible individuals. She noted that CMS recently released a regulation that requires social needs screening for people that are dually eligible. She added that Medicare continues to partner with Medicaid to find opportunities to develop better aligned infrastructure to support care for people that are dually enrolled. Reuben noted that not everybody with ADRD is eligible to enroll in both Medicare and Medicaid because many people have an income that is just above the level that would allow them to be eligible for Medicaid. He added that funding gaps can be particularly problematic for those individuals. Reuben noted that additional research will be needed to determine the most effective approach for funding ADRD care and support provided by community-based organizations.

Sarah Lenz Lock, AARP and the Global Council on Brain Health, noted that most people with ADRD present to their health care providers with other comorbidities that their health care provider may prioritize over managing ADRD. She asked if addressing the cognitive and behavioral issues related to the patient's ADRD before addressing other comorbidities could improve quality of care. Dr. Reuben explained that specialty care for those comorbidities, such as diabetes, hypertension, or chronic obstructive pulmonary disease (COPD) is important because it decreases the likelihood of hospitalization for people with ADRD. He added that those providers often lack the resources and expertise to adequately address ADRD. He noted this highlights the importance of coordinated dementia care models.

3

Defining Quality

Terry Fulmer, The John A. Hartford Foundation (JAHF) and session moderator, noted in her introduction that identifying optimal approaches to facilitate systemic change to improve the quality of care for people with Alzheimer's disease and related dementia (ADRD) will require collaboration among all organizations engaged in research efforts. Fulmer cited several JAHF initiatives to illustrate opportunities for foundations to collaborate with the National Institute on Aging (NIA), the Centers for Disease Control and Prevention (CDC), and health care systems to accelerate innovation for improving the quality of care for people with ADRD. These initiatives include

- dissemination and implementation of the evidence-based 4 Ms framework (what *m*atters, *m*edication, *m*entation, and *m*obility)[1] in 2,900 geriatric care settings;
- improvement in emergency care with geriatric emergency department (GED) accreditation and a GED collaborative;
- a geriatric surgical verification program (Hwang et al., 2022);

---

[1] What matters: understanding an individual patient's health goals and care preferences across settings and aligning care (including but not limited to end-of-life care) with those goals and preferences. Medication: if medication is necessary, using age-friendly medications that do not hamper the other 3 Ms. Mentation: preventing, identifying, treating, and managing dementia, depression, and delirium across care settings. Mobility: ensuring older people move safely daily to sustain function and do the things identified in what matters (JAF, 2018).

- the recently released National Academies of Sciences, Engineering, and Medicine consensus study report, *The National Imperative to Improve Nursing Home Quality*;
- the UCLA Alzheimer's and Dementia Care Program;
- Best Practice Caregiving,[2] which provides free online resources to assist organizations and consumers to select evidence-based programs that support family caregivers; and
- the Milken Institute Alliance to Improve Dementia Care (NASEM, 2022).[3]

THE NATIONAL IMPERATIVE TO IMPROVE NURSING HOME QUALITY

Betty Ferrell, City of Hope, began the session with a discussion of the National Academies of Sciences, Engineering, and Medicine 2022 consensus study report, *The National Imperative to Improve Nursing Home Quality: Honoring Our Commitment to Residents, Families, and Staff*. Ferrell, who was the committee chair for the consensus study, explained that the project sought to "examine how our nation delivers, regulates, finances, and measures the quality of nursing home care [and] delineate a framework and general principles for improving the quality of care in nursing homes" (NASEM, 2022). The committee envisioned nursing home quality as follows: "Residents of nursing homes should receive care in a safe environment that honors their values and preferences, addresses goals of care, promotes equity, and assesses the benefits and risks of care and treatment" (NASEM, 2022). The consensus report included a robust discussion of inequities in nursing home care and noted that quality improvement measures must not exacerbate existing disparities. The development of the report included an 18-month process of weighing evidence and consulting with experts, family members of people residing in nursing homes, and residents of nursing homes. She said that the committee's first conclusion was that the United States' current approach to financing and delivering care in nursing homes "is ineffective, inefficient, fragmented, and unsustainable" (NASEM, 2022). Another conclusion noted the need for high-quality research to address quality-of-care issues. The committee also found that underinvestment in mechanisms to ensure quality of care and a lack of accountability related to resource allocation have had a negative effect on the nursing home sector.

Ferrell (with assistance from Terry Fulmer, due to technical issues) briefly described each of the report's seven key goals that provide a framework for

---

[2] See https://bpc.caregiver.org/#home (accessed July 26, 2022).
[3] See https://milkeninstitute.org/centers/center-for-the-future-of-aging/alliance-to-improve-dementia-care (accessed September 28, 2022).

improving quality of care in nursing homes and highlighted pertinent recommendations for achieving those goals (a more detailed discussion of the consensus report goals and recommendations can be found in that report). The first goal is for nursing homes to provide care that is comprehensive, person centered, and equitable; ensures residents' health, quality of life, and safety; promotes autonomy; and manages risks (NASEM, 2022). Recommendations to achieve this goal address care planning, models of care, emergency preparedness, and the physical environment. The second goal connects to the previous workshop discussion about the caregiving workforce. That goal is to ensure that the nursing home workforce is well prepared, empowered, and appropriately compensated (NASEM, 2022). She noted that this is essential for the delivery of high-quality care. Recommendations to achieve this goal emphasize competitive wages and benefits, staffing standards, empowering skilled nursing assistants, education and training, data collection, and research.

The third goal is to increase the transparency and accountability of nursing home finances, operations, and ownership (NASEM, 2022). A key recommendation for this goal is to collect, audit, and report detailed facility-level data. That data should be publicly available and easily searchable. The fourth goal is to develop a more "rational, robust financing system," with a recommendation for research into establishing a federal long-term care benefit as well as exploring broader application of other alternative payment models, such as bundled payment (NASEM, 2022). The fifth goal is to design an effective and responsive system of quality assurance. Recommendations to achieve this goal address CMS oversight and support of state nursing home surveys as well as improved transparency and accountability (NASEM, 2022).

The sixth goal is to expand and enhance quality measurement and continuous quality improvement. Recommendations related to this goal call for improved measures of resident and family experience; enhancement and expansion of Care Compare; development and adoption of new quality measures; development of health equity strategies; as well as technical assistance for quality improvement (NASEM, 2022). The seventh goal is to adopt health information technology (HIT) in all nursing homes. Recommendations consider pathways to provide financial incentives for electronic health record (EHR) adoption; measures of HIT adoption and interoperability; perceptions of HIT usability; and training in core HIT competencies (NASEM, 2022).

Ferrell explained that the findings and recommendations included in the study also apply to improving quality of care for people with ADRD that reside in nursing homes. She added that the implications of the findings in the study should be regarded with an additional sense of urgency when considering how to best meet the needs of patients with ADRD. Since the report's release in April 2022, members of the consensus study committee have presented the report's conclusions and recommendations to several congressional committees and policy makers at all levels of government. They have also discussed the report with members of the media and members of the general public. She noted that these interactions have elicited a uniformly positive response, which highlights the importance of prompt action on the report's findings.

DEFINING QUALITY

Dr. Eric Schneider is a health disparities researcher who now leads digital quality transformation at the National Committee for Quality Assurance (NCQA). NCQA accredits health plans and home- and community-based organizations, offers recognition programs for patient-centered medical homes and diabetes care, and provides awards of distinction that are awarded to health insurers that meet those standards. He contributed to the development of NCQA's Healthcare Effectiveness Data and Information Set (HEDIS) performance measurement system,[4] which was primarily developed for health insurers, and has since been repurposed for application to diabetes, cardiovascular disease, medication management, and other topics.

Schneider began with a personal story that illustrated several of the challenges that people with ADRD and their families can encounter in the health care system. His stepmother was living in an independent living community when the COVID-19 pandemic began. Over time she lost the ability to participate in video calls, which were her primary source of social interaction. Her condition continued to worsen, which resulted in her being transferred to the independent living community's personal care unit. She then received numerous treatments for delirium, including medication, hospitalizations, and rehabilitation over the course of several months. However, she did not receive a full neurological evaluation until her delirium resolved and her worsened memory became more apparent. Schneider explained that he had observed patients and their families encounter similar experiences several times in his practice as a primary care physician. He noted that navigating the experience in the role of caregiver provided him with a new perspective.

Schneider explained that this experience illustrated several quality-of-care issues encountered by people with ADRD and their families. The first issue was that early stages of memory loss may not be noticeable to facility staff, which can lead to staff framing ADRD behavioral symptoms as intentional rather than a manifestation of the disease. Schneider noted that another issue was that his observations were frequently disregarded by facility staff. Additionally, he said the difficulties encountered while attempting to obtain a neuropsychiatric evaluation for his stepmother illustrated the urgent need to increase access to specialty care in rural areas. He also emphasized that when a person has a diagnosis of ADRD, proper and adaptive medication management is critical.

---

[4] See https://www.ncqa.org/hedis/ (accessed on June 7, 2022).

Schneider said his stepmother's experiences also highlighted the need for improved coordination of care for people with ADRD. The conceptual model from the National Academies *National Imperative to Improve Nursing Home Quality* (Figure 3-1) presents a well-structured quality model but is organization specific. He said that organization-specific quality models usually are not designed to address issues outside of the target organization. This includes areas that affect the quality of care for people with ADRD, such as gaps in coordination of care that extend outside of the institution, such as obtaining a primary care physician, accessing specialty care, and understanding health insurance coverage. This coordination occurs *between* organizations such as insurers, care delivery organizations, public health agencies, social service agencies, and community-based organizations, all of which interact with patients and caregivers. He noted that from the patient's perspective, the root of gaps in quality of care originates with inadequate coordination among organizations and clinicians. This could be addressed through an approach similar to the patient-centered medical home that has been used to improve quality in primary care.

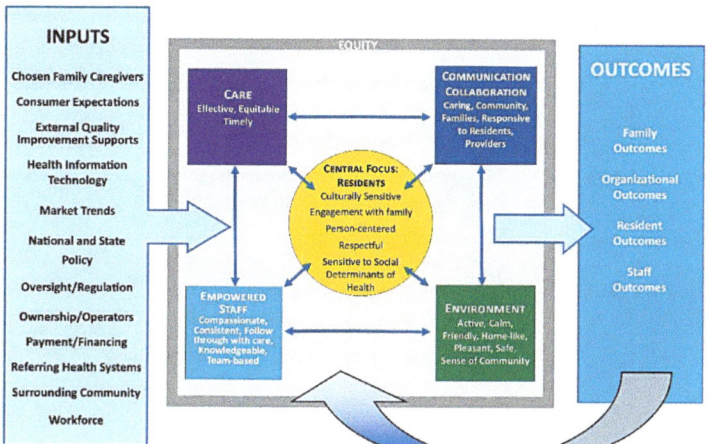

FIGURE 3-1 National Academies consensus study conceptual model of quality of care in nursing homes.
SOURCE: Presented by Eric Schneider, May 23, 2022, at Mechanisms for Organizational Behavior Change to Address the Needs of People Living with Alzheimer's Disease and Related Dementias: A Workshop. Reproduced from National Academies of Sciences, Engineering, and Medicine. 2022. *The National Imperative to Improve Nursing home quality: Honoring our commitment to residents, families, and staff.* Washington, DC: The National Academies Press. https://doi.org/10.17226/26526.

Schneider provided an example of one such model that is centered on a stepwise approach to implementation (Figure 3-2). This approach begins with a foundation of a quality improvement strategy and engaged leadership. Then, each step requires specific fundamental components, such as empanelment and continuous and team-based healing relationships, to be in place before progressing to the next step. All of the fundamental components of the model must be in place to result in reduced barriers to care through improved access and coordination of care (Wagner et al., 2014).

Schneider proposed several accountability imperatives for the quality of care for people with ADRD. He described the first imperative, situational awareness, as the capability of all participants in the care of a person with ADRD to exchange data quickly so problems can be identified more quickly. Most quality measurement systems have relied on insurance claims data, which are usually reported several months after the episode of care and may not

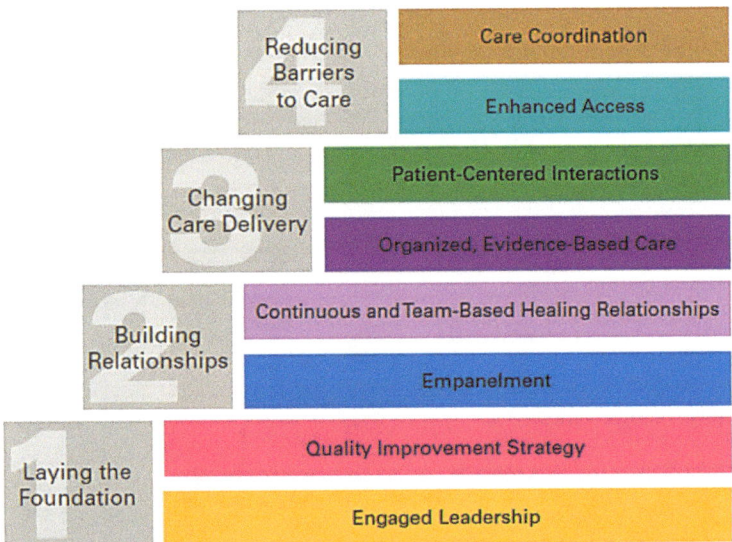

FIGURE 3-2 Stepwise development of capabilities for the patient-centered medical home.
SOURCE: Presented by Eric Schneider, May 23, 2022, at Mechanisms for Organizational Behavior Change to Address the Needs of People Living with Alzheimer's Disease and Related Dementias: A Workshop. Reprinted from *Primary Care: Clinics in Office Practice*, Vol. 39 Issue 2, Wagner, E. H., K. Coleman, R. J. Reid, K. Phillips, M. K. Abrams, J. R. Sugarman, The Changes Involved in Patient-Centered Medical Home Transformation, pp. 241-259, Copyright 2012, with permission from Elsevier.

include specific date and time information. That creates challenges for using these data to understand a sequence of events. Schneider emphasized that care coordination and effective communication among all involved are necessary. He noted this becomes particularly crucial as patients with ADRD experience disease progression, which can result in multiple transitions in where a patient lives and receives care. Quality metrics must be thoughtfully designed to avoid creating incentives for staff caring for patients with ADRD to act in ways that are counterproductive for the patient's well-being. He offered an example of a quality metric for fall prevention that leads to staff reprimanding patients for standing up from their chairs. Data should be obtained on intermediate health outcomes, such as functional status, cognitive ability, and behavioral symptoms instead of prioritizing end-state outcomes. Quality measurement systems should also integrate care goal attainment in addition to the commonly used clinical measures, he said.

Schneider noted that the more timely and robust data exchange that he described requires improvements in the existing health care data infrastructure. NCQA is focused on expanding the use of electronic data in order to improve the information available for quality measurement. This work has gained momentum following passage of the 21st Century Cures Act,[5] updated data exchange and interoperability regulations, and federal broadband investments. Schneider cautioned that while changing payment incentives is fundamentally necessary, additional strategies and investments may be necessary to attain needed digital infrastructure updates, systems reengineering, and other organizational changes.

QUALITY IN ADVANCED ADRD CARE TRANSITIONS

Lisa Gwyther, Duke School of Medicine and founder of the Duke Aging Center's Dementia Family Support Program, discussed her experience navigating acute care transitions as a family caregiver with expertise in quality care for people with ADRD. Gwyther's husband, Bob, a retired clinician and professor of family medicine, has advanced Lewy body dementia.

Gwyther described the quality indicators and systemic issues she observed when Bob experienced two transitions from a skilled nursing facility to different hospitals, one week apart, due to acute respiratory distress. During the first care transition, Gwyther and her husband experienced several benefits of

---

[5] See https://www.congress.gov/bill/114th-congress/house-bill/34 and https://www.federalregister.gov/documents/2020/08/04/C2-2020-07419/21st-century-cures-act-interoperability-information-blocking-and-the-onc-health-it-certification (both accessed September 29, 2022).

systems that were designed to be dementia friendly. When the care transition occurred, a geriatrician on call at the skilled nursing facility recommended transfer to a hospital that had completed specific steps to be classified as dementia friendly. When Gwyther arrived at the hospital and explained to staff that her husband had dementia and could not be left unattended, she was quickly able to join her husband in the emergency department (ED). The staff at the dementia-friendly hospital had received specific training to support the unique needs of patients with ADRD and their family caregivers. The attending physician in the ED suggested that Gwyther consider completing a medical order for scope of treatment (MOST) form for end-of-life planning.[6] When Bob returned to the skilled nursing facility, the speech therapist there observed Gwyther feeding Bob and posted notes for staff about how to help him eat and drink safely.

Gwyther also encountered several barriers to effective treatment for her husband during the first episode of care transitions. The ambulance emergency medical technicians (EMTs) initially resisted Gwyther's hospital choice and argued for taking her husband to the closer academic medical center. Bob had to spend 3 days under NPO (nothing by mouth) orders while waiting for a swallowing evaluation because of procedural regulations and staff shortages at the hospital.

The second care transition from the skilled nursing facility to an ED illustrated several systemic problems that negatively affected quality of care. The ambulance EMTs took Bob to the nearby academic medical center ED, despite the MOST form on file at the skilled nursing facility and Gwyther's wishes. Gwyther and her husband were kept separated at the ED for several hours due to that hospital's COVID-19 protocols, which were not specifically designed in a dementia-friendly manner. When Lisa was able to join Bob in the ED, he was visibly upset. Gwyther then spent the next 12 hours negotiating a transfer to a dementia-friendly hospital, where he was later discharged 8 hours after admission.

Gwyther described several lessons learned through her experiences that could inform quality care for people with ADRD:

- The goals and preferences of the patient and family change depending on the circumstances.
- Clinicians should incorporate the family as a resource for understanding the patient's goals, especially during care transitions.

---

[6] See https://www.kymost.org/most-form-v2 (accessed on July 7, 2022).

- Quality dementia care should be led by clinicians and direct-care staff with geriatric and dementia-specific skills.
- Cordial, practiced working relationships between hospital discharge planners and skilled nursing facility clinicians are needed to ensure quality, safe transfers.
- Existing systems, structures, and protocols (such as an insistence on taking a patient with ADRD to the nearest hospital) may unintentionally negatively affect the quality of care for people with ADRD.
- Constant communication, checking mutual understandings, and timely action are keys to quality in dementia care transitions.

DISCUSSION

Lessons from Lived Experiences

Terry Fulmer began the discussion by asking Ferrell to reflect on Gwyther's and Schneider's experiences in relation to the National Academies nursing home consensus study. Ferrell began by noting that patients with ADRD frequently encounter disconnects in medical care. Those issues are often exacerbated without a family caregiver to advocate on the patient's behalf. Ferrell explained that the nursing home consensus study report emphasized that quality care initiatives should begin by identifying the people who would be affected by those initiatives and considering how those initiatives would affect those people's quality of life. She added that efforts to develop a model to improve quality of care for people with ADRD should ensure that quality care is not limited to those patients with the greatest resources. Schneider noted that despite relatively good circumstances, the dedicated and compassionate staff were unable to coordinate care across systems for Gwyther's husband. He added that these challenges highlight the need for reengineering the health care ecosystem to reduce current fragmentation.

Schneider suggested that electronic data could be used for early detection of problems. Credit card companies rapidly identify irregular patterns that could indicate a problem such as fraud. Patient portal applications, such as MyChart, have the capability to send alerts to users. He suggested that if health care systems had a similar data monitoring and interpretation system in place to detect abnormalities, it could speed the delivery of appropriate care to address that issue. He noted that a patient being placed on NPO status for 3 days is an example of an abnormality that should raise an alert in an EHR just as unusual charges would raise an alert with a credit card company.

Gwyther said that while navigating a relative through dementia care is challenging, caregiver expectations should incorporate an understanding of the challenging circumstances health care workers often encounter while providing care for people with ADRD. She added that having a caregiver who knows the patient well and a comprehensive care team can have a positive effect on quality of care. Fulmer highlighted the importance of personal stories, such as Gwyther's and Schneider's, in communicating the necessity of systemic change to improve the quality of care for people with ADRD to multiple audiences.

Reframing Reliance on EDs

Several participants noted that, in the current system, ED visits have become central to the care of individuals with ADRD. Vladeck explained that EDs are generally not ideal care settings for people with ADRD. He added that frequently the hospital ED where a patient with ADRD is transported to does not have a relationship with the physicians that manage the person's care. He suggested that reducing reliance on EDs could be translated into a measurable quality-of-care indicator.

Culturally Responsive Quality

Faith Mitchell, Urban Institute, noted the disproportionately high rates of ADRD in the Black population, who have historically experienced health inequity. She added that most quality-of-care recommendations do not specifically address the contributors to that inequity, such as inadequate access, distrust, and language barriers. She asked how the discussion of strategies to improve quality of care could be better translated to more specifically address quality of care for people with ADRD that have experienced chronic health inequities.

Ferrell noted that health equity is integrated throughout the goals and recommendations in the National Academies of Sciences, Engineering, and Medicine consensus study report. Quality care should integrate culturally responsive care. Ferrell added that culturally responsive care requires practitioner training, and a strong recommendation of the report was to hold nursing homes accountable for this training. Schneider noted that NCQA is launching a redesigned health equity accreditation program. He explained that efforts to develop quality measures to address issues of distrust and unequal treatment should include engagement with communities. Schneider described the example of West Side United,[7] a community-based organization in Chicago that collaborated with seven hospitals serving the people that live and work

---

[7] See https://westsideunited.org/ (accessed September 29, 2022).

on the West Side of Chicago to identify key quality indicators and create joint accountability.

The Relationship Among Staffing, Training, Pay, and Care

Schneider remarked that at the time of the workshop, 30 to 40 of the staff at his stepmother's skilled nursing facility were not at work because of COVID-19 infection, and he added that these settings were already understaffed and experienced high rates of staff turnover before the pandemic. He asked fellow participants to discuss possible approaches to address staffing issues in facilities that care for people with ADRD. Ferrell noted that the high nationwide rate of COVID-19 infections among nursing home staff are illustrative of broader safety issues in the industry. She explained that the high staff turnover rates in nursing homes affects quality of care and health equity because staff are less familiar with each resident and that person's values and preferences. Staff compensation affects the ability to attract and retain qualified nursing home staff.

Ferrell also discussed the need to harness innovations in technology to develop quality, nationally disseminated training programs for nursing home staff. She emphasized that addressing core issues of staff pay, training, and retention is necessary to achieve improved quality of care. Several participants also noted the effects of labor shortages, most notably in nursing, on quality of care for people living with ADRD. Peter Hollmann, Brown University, noted the need to recognize the importance of long-term care, and the need to treat the people that work in that field as professionals. He opined that the nursing shortage is one of the most significant crises facing the United States.

Hollmann explained that fragmentation of the health care system has created substantial barriers for a patient care team to effectively cross care settings. He added that it is likely that a patient with ADRD who has been transferred several times among different care settings has also had to begin care with a new care team with each transfer. Gwyther added that this highlights the importance of a comprehensive, coordinated, and consistent care team that "becomes an expert in that individual" to improve quality of care for people with ADRD. She suggested that examples of quality team-based care can be used in training and scaled up from small settings. Schneider said quality care for people with ADRD should foster a team-based model of care that includes community caregivers along with professionals; provide training in these interactions; and disincentivize the adversarial relationship that can develop between different sectors when they are caring for people with ADRD.

Strategies to Reduce Stigma

Fulmer asked speakers to comment on the role of ageism in existing barriers to quality of care for people with ADRD. Gwyther noted, "I think that people think of older people as less interesting, less complicated than they really are, and less diverse than they really are." She added that the Gerontological Society of America is working to reframe aging in a manner that is less stigmatizing, less discriminatory, and recognizes the diversity of the aging experience. Sarah Lenz Lock, AARP and Global Brain Health Initiative and a speaker in a later session of the workshop, suggested that education and training for younger health care providers may offer an opportunity to address some issues related to ageism. Those providers and their patients will benefit if the provider understands how to have conversations with patients about their priorities. Those providers should also understand that while ADRD does not currently have a cure, some challenges associated with the disease can be effectively addressed.

Fulmer noted the collaboration between JAHF and the Institute for Healthcare Improvement (IHI) on age-friendly health systems. A key component of that work is to center care on the 4 Ms—what *m*atters, *m*entation, *m*edication, and *m*obility, specific to each patient. Ferrell added that including social workers as part of the care team for patients with ADRD is helpful because they have skills and training to directly interact with patients and ensure that their identity and needs are preserved across the care continuum. She emphasized that high-quality care provided by qualified people in a safe environment is possible for people with ADRD, and family members should have that expectation. Sharon Inouye added that conversations about improving quality of care for people with ADRD are often accompanied by fear, hopelessness, and a sense of inevitability that create a sense of inertia around creating change. She noted that while this is a complex problem, there are many possible solutions, but that inertia must be overcome.

Creative Solutions for Quality Care

Elisabeth Belmont, MaineHealth and planning committee member, asked for speakers' perspectives on the most effective payment model to promote quality care for people with ADRD. Schneider noted that the health care system is transitioning from fee-for-service reimbursement models to value-based contracting. That transition is another reason to ensure quality measurement systems are well designed. He cautioned against overestimating the improvements that could be achieved through an approach that relies only on financial incentives. He encouraged participants to consider approaches that incorporate infrastructure improvements and direct payments.

Julie Robison, University of Connecticut School of Medicine and planning committee member, noted that emergency medical service (EMS) companies, whose providers respond to 911 calls, are usually not reimbursed for care provided unless they transport the patient to a hospital. She asked speakers to share their thoughts about training EMS staff to provide care to people with ADRD in the patient's home and changing reimbursement rules to support that approach. Schneider noted that he believed there were organizations that were investigating this approach. Fulmer described the variety of care providers and community organizations that could collaborate to provide care and support for people with ADRD and their caregivers. She offered an example from her home town in upstate New York. In that small town, if there is a significant staff shortage at the local hospital, the National Guard provides patient care. She added that while it can be unnerving to see the National Guard at the health care facility, they provide excellent care. Fulmer explained that in small towns, the first responder to a 911 call is usually a firefighter, who also lives in that town. Those local first responders are usually familiar with the people in their town who have a memory problem. Fulmer suggested that conversations about coordination of care for people with ADRD should include first responders. She added that another opportunity for collaboration is with community organizations, such as YMCAs and libraries, that are resources for adult day programs for people in preclinical or mild stages of ADRD. She emphasized that the United States has large infrastructures in place that could collaborate to improve care and support for people with ADRD, their families, and caregivers.

Schneider noted that caregivers should not be overlooked as sources of innovation because they often must find creative solutions to problems encountered when caring for a person with ADRD. He cited an example of an engineer who had a family member with health issues who used inexpensive components to create a motion detection system to alert the family to problems. Schneider suggested increasing support for caregiver innovations. Fulmer added that Japan, which has a dearth of young people relative to its older adult population, innovates with robotics. She also recommended participants review a recent World Health Organization (WHO) framework developed to help countries strengthen their long-term care systems and services (WHO, 2021).

4

Transforming the Role of Payment System Incentives to Improve Quality

OPPORTUNITIES TO ALIGN PAYMENT WITH IMPROVING CARE FOR ALZHEIMER'S DISEASE

Tisamarie Sherry, deputy assistant secretary for Behavioral Health, Disability, and Aging Policy in the U.S. Department of Health and Human Services (HHS) Office of the Assistant Secretary for Planning and Evaluation (ASPE), discussed the payment landscape for people with ADRD; how this influences care delivery and quality; and promising payment models. The Office of Behavioral Health, Disability, and Aging Policy coordinates dementia care, research, and policy and oversees implementation of the National Alzheimer's Project Act, which maintains the National Plan to Address Alzheimer's Disease.

Sherry said that two-thirds of people living with ADRD live at home and receive care and services in their home from home health workers and unpaid family caregivers, as well as care in ambulatory care (outpatient) settings. The care settings for the remaining one-third of people with ADRD are approximately evenly divided between nursing homes and other supportive settings, such as assisted living facilities (Chi et al., 2019). Ninety-five percent of these individuals are enrolled in Medicare, and 24 percent have dual Medicare/Medicaid eligibility (Garfield et al., 2015). Nonetheless, families pay 70 percent of the lifetime expenditures for ADRD care in the form of out-of-pocket care expenses and unpaid caregiving (Jutkowitz et al., 2017).

She explained that the two public payers, Medicare and Medicaid, cover different types of ADRD care and services. Medicare pays for ambulatory care, hospital care, post-acute care, physical therapy (PT) and occupational therapy (OT), and hospice care. Medicaid's major role is in financing long-term nursing home stays as well as home- and community-based services (HCBS). Medicaid also serves as a payer of last resort for hospital and ambulatory care.[1] Care settings and payers change over the course of ADRD progression. As people with ADRD age and their disease progresses, more of those people transition from residing at home to institutional settings. Seventy-five percent of people over age 80 with ADRD reside in nursing homes (Alzheimer's Association, 2022). Medicaid becomes the dominant source of reimbursement for care for people with ADRD as they exhaust their financial resources.

Sherry noted that the features of our current payment system have a number of implications for ADRD care and the quality of that care. Payment is typically tied to specific clinical settings. This creates complications for coordination of care as people transition among care settings (e.g., from hospital to skilled nursing facility). It also creates a funding gap for care provided in a patient's home, where most people living with ADRD actually receive care and prefer to receive care (Grabowski, 2007; NASEM, 2022). She explained that there is also fragmentation in care across payers, which contributes to challenges in coordinating person-centered care for patients with ADRD and aligning incentives across the two public payers. For example, Medicaid covers long-term nursing home care, whereas Medicare, which typically has a higher reimbursement rate for care, covers hospital and post-acute care. This creates a condition in which nursing homes are incentivized to send long-term residents to the hospital in order to receive Medicare's higher reimbursement rate for care provided at the nursing home upon the patient's return to the nursing home because that can be categorized as post-acute care.

Sherry explained that while state Medicaid plans are required to cover nursing homes, coverage of HCBS is optional. Therefore, Medicaid-supported HCBS programs often have multiple barriers to access, such as stringent qualification requirements; limited enrollment capacity, which often leads to lengthy waiting lists; and time limitations (Johnson and Lindner, 2016; Ryan and Edwards, 2015). She noted that over the last few decades, rebalancing efforts from institutional care to HCBS and the increasing number of assisted living facilities have gradually decreased the number of people with Medicare or private insurance residing in nursing homes. This has combined with a more recent pandemic-related decline in patients seeking facility-based post-acute care to contribute to a shift in the populations of patients residing in nursing homes toward more patients that rely on Medicaid. Those patients also often have more complex medical needs, but their care is reimbursed at a lower rate than that of a patient covered by Medicare or private insurance (Cornell et al., 2020; Werner and Bressman, 2021). She added that over time this has resulted in nursing

---

[1] See https://www.cms.gov/Outreach-and-Education/American-Indian-Alaska-Native/AIAN/LTSS-TA-Center/info/hcbs (accessed July 25, 2022).

homes caring for more complicated patients, but having fewer resources with which to provide that care.

Sherry noted that receiving a timely ADRD diagnosis is important for planning as well as access to therapy and clinical trials. However, fewer than half of the people living with ADRD receive a physician's diagnosis, particularly in the early stages of disease (Lang et al., 2017; NASEM, 2022; Savva and Arthur, 2015). Health care providers have cited payment-related barriers to early diagnosis, such as insufficient time in their clinical workflow to perform cognitive assessments (Korthauer et al., 2021). Another challenge for people with ADRD is difficulty transitioning between care settings. People living with ADRD, particularly those with unmet caregiver needs, are at higher risk of readmission and mortality following hospitalization (Anderson et al., 2022; Knox et al., 2020a, 2020b). She explained that while providing caregiver support and home-based support for people living with ADRD during care transitions is beneficial, the gap in financing for these services makes this difficult. Patients with ADRD will have increasing care needs as their disease progresses. However, their caregivers often face burnout (Hiyoshi-Taniguchi et al., 2018).

The home-based care financing gap creates barriers to supplementing family caregivers with additional paid caregivers. The course of ADRD does not fit the trajectory of the Medicare hospice benefit for end-of-life care. The life span of those with late-stage ADRD can be difficult to predict. Additionally, Medicare disenrollment rates are high among patients with late-stage ADRD. This suggests that the Medicare hospice benefit frequently does not meet these patients' needs (De Vleminck et al., 2018). The combined effect of the payment landscape and the clinical features of ADRD leads to a substantial reliance on unpaid caregivers, high out-of-pocket spending, and increased reliance on Medicaid-financed nursing home care.

Sherry cited three elements of payment models that have shown promise for ADRD care:

- Person-centered payment, which follows the patient across care settings (Boustani et al., 2019);
- Improved integration and coordination across payers to better align incentives for quality improvement (NASEM, 2022); and
- Value-based payment, including both accountability for quality and the flexibility to reimburse for valuable services that are not typically covered by traditional insurance, such as caregiver training and community-based supports.

Sherry described current payment tools that could support integrating those elements (Table 4-1). These include adding value-based payment incentives to existing setting-specific payment schemes, such as the Medicare Merit-

TABLE 4-1 Existing Payment Models That Include Elements with Promise to Improve Quality of Care for People with ADRD

Value-Based Payment, Setting Specific	Medicare Merit-Based Incentive Payment System Medicaid Value-Based Payment Programs for Nursing Homes
Value-Based Payment	Medicare Shared Savings Program
Person-Centered with some Long-Term Services and Supports (LTSS) Elements	Medicare Advantage (MA) Institutional Special Needs Plans (I-SNPs) MA expanded primarily health-related supplemental benefits MA Special Supplemental Benefits for the Chronically Ill (SSBCI) Medicaid Managed LTSS Medicaid Consumer Self-Direction Medicaid Money Follows the Person
Person-Centered, Coordinated Across Payers	CMS Financial Alignment Initiative Duel-Eligible SNPs (D-SNPs), Fully/Highly Integrated D-SNPs Program of All-Inclusive Care for the Elderly (PACE)
End-of-Life Care	MA Value-BasedInsurance Design (VBID) Hospice Benefit

SOURCE: Presented by Tisamarie Sherry on May 23, 2022 the workshop Mechanisms for Organizational Behavior Change to Address the Needs of People Living with Alzheimer's Disease and Related Dementias.

based Incentive Payment System and value-based incentives that coordinate care across settings, such as the Medicare Shared Savings Program.

Other opportunities include existing person-centered payment models, some of which offer support for long-term care, such as Medicaid Managed Long-Term Services and Supports (LTSS). Some models also reimburse services from unpaid family caregivers, such as Medicaid Consumer Self-Direction HCBS waivers. She also noted current person-centered models, which are primarily directed at individuals that are dually eligible that coordinate across payers. CMS is also currently evaluating the Medicare Advantage Value-Based Insurance Design (VBID) Hospice Benefit for end-of-life care.

Sherry next described several research needs to determine how to better align payment policy with quality and outcomes for the care of people living with ADRD. More evidence is needed about the effects of value-based payment or integrated care programs (with the exception of the Program of All-Inclusive Care for the Elderly [PACE])[2] on outcomes for people with ADRD (Feng et al., 2021). There is also little evidence on the role of payment in quality of care in assisted living facilities. She added that while care provided in assisted living facilities is less affected by public funding models because that

---

[2] Program of All-inclusive Care for the Elderly, see: https://www.cms.gov/Medicare-Medicaid-Coordination/Medicare-and-Medicaid-Coordination/Medicare-Medicaid-Coordination-Office/PACE/PACE (accessed September 29, 2022).

care is mostly funded by private insurers, those patients receive hospital and ambulatory care that is paid for by Medicare. Many of those patients will transition to relying on Medicaid to pay for their care. States would also benefit from more evidence to guide Medicaid HCBS program design. This includes investigating how the various HCBS waiver designs influence the delivery of quality care and outcomes for people with ADRD (Wang et al., 2020). She also highlighted the need to evaluate the effects of different payment models on equitable access and treatment, particularly for people with ADRD from historically marginalized communities (NASEM, 2022). Additional research is also needed to identify which payment models are most likely to improve the quality of end-of-life care for people with ADRD.

Sherry noted that reforming the payment system is not sufficient to improve quality of care for people with ADRD. While the PACE model contains many of the desired elements for delivery of quality ADRD care, its uptake has been limited in part by high regulatory barriers. Medicare adopted Cognitive Assessment and Care Plan billing codes in 2017 to incentivize providers to perform a cognitive assessment during a patient's annual wellness exam, which should improve the rate of early diagnosis. However, the increase in cognitive assessments has been much lower than anticipated (Li et al., 2021). Sherry said a key research need is to determine the optimal combination of payment, delivery system, and regulatory changes.

PAYMENT MODELS FOR POPULATIONS WITH SPECIAL NEEDS

Amol Navathe, associate director of the Penn Center for Health Incentives and Behavioral Economics at University of Pennsylvania, began by noting that patients with ADRD are a population with special needs. His presentation offered a conceptual grounding for selecting among existing payment models for special needs populations. He organized existing payment models into four categories:

1. Episode-based, which is primarily focused on episodes of care in the hospital or specialty care setting;
2. Population-based, such as accountable care organizations (ACOs) or shared savings programs that manage all care for a population;
3. Full capitation, as used in Medicare Advantage; and
4. Comprehensive primary care, which is designed to motivate innovation in primary care for patients with high needs.

Navathe said that none of these models adequately meets the needs of patients with ADRD. This is largely because people living with ADRD have unique, relatively intense, and longitudinal care needs over the course of their disease. He added that research evidence to support any of those models for financing ADRD care is very limited.

Navathe explained that patients with ADRD receive a combination of non-ADRD- and ADRD-specific care, and it is important not to conflate the two. There is evidence on how some payment models affect non-ADRD care for conditions that are not uncommon to patients with ADRD. Research findings have demonstrated that bundled payment models for medical conditions, such as congestive heart failure, maintained the quality of care for vulnerable individuals, and participation in an ACO was associated with fewer hospitalizations among individuals living in long-term care (Chang et al., 2021; Maughan et al., 2019). However, few studies examine how these models affect the longitudinal, ADRD-related care and disease trajectory of individuals with ADRD. Initial consideration of that question has revealed notable challenges.

He described a study that suggested ACOs may avoid patients with ADRD due to the intensity of spending and care, and this bias can interact with racial, social, and ethnic disparities (Chang et al., 2019). While evidence suggests that there may be better end-of-life care for patients with ADRD enrolled in Medicare Advantage plans, such as fewer deaths in-hospital and less mechanical ventilation, this is counterbalanced by concerns around selection. The population of patients with ADRD also presents technical challenges in areas such as risk adjustment. Navathe urged researchers and clinicians to recognize that changes in payment models affect ADRD care and non-ADRD care differently, even within the same population. Navathe explained that in earlier efforts, changing payments did not yield the desired changes in organizational models. He suggested that instead of starting with payments, change efforts should begin by examining the organizational model and considering how to best deliver care in the context of that model. Organizational models that promote high-quality ADRD care should incorporate support for caregivers, medication management, self-management, psychosocial interventions, and longitudinality.

Navathe noted that salience is a challenge for population health payment models. Salience in this case refers to the need to engage clinicians that are providing adequate care to people living with ADRD. Engaging these physicians requires a model that is specialized but not overly engineered. Navathe suggested a baseline population payment model approach, which would invest in care infrastructure, supplemented with episodic care. This approach would establish a payment baseline with additional reimbursement for episodic care. The model could be tailored to the needs of individuals with ADRD but salient enough to engage providers in redesigning care to incorporate disease-specific elements. Navathe cautioned that more research is needed to establish a strong link between payment models and organizational care delivery.

SYSTEMIC CONSIDERATIONS FOR IMPROVING QUALITY OF CARE AND SUPPORT FOR PEOPLE WITH ADRD AND THEIR CAREGIVERS

Bruce Vladeck, senior advisor to the Greater New York Hospital Association and LiveOnNY, began by emphasizing that in order to improve care for people with ADRD, reform efforts should go beyond payment policy. He argued that the notion of payment system incentives reflects an exaggerated view of the ability of payment mechanisms to actually affect the way care is delivered. Vladeck was struck by Reuben's comment that "hospitals don't get paid for adoption [of the UCLA Alzheimer's and Dementia Care Model]." He explained that hospitals could use funds they receive from Medicare to implement care models such as the UCLA Alzheimer's and Dementia Care Model. Medicare pays hospitals a lump sum that is based on a patient's diagnosis and complications. That money is allocated at the discretion of the hospital, provided it meets regulatory and professional standards. The hospital, for example, could choose to use some of those funds to support employing a nurse practitioner to manage care coordination for patients with ADRD. He suggested that payment in terms of adequate reimbursement may not be a barrier to changing patterns of care for patients with ADRD. Payment under the current model may serve as an incentive for hospitals to change patterns of care for people with ADRD in some areas, such as reducing their length of stay in the hospital.

Vladeck explained that there are three dimensions to consider when determining how to reimburse for care and services. The three dimensions are the source of payment (who pays), the amount of payment (how much is paid), and the payment mechanism (how providers are paid). He suggested that the overall health care system and individual health care organizations should give greater consideration to payment mechanisms, particularly in reference to care for patients with ADRD. Currently, Medicaid reimbursement is the primary public payment mechanism for long-term care. He noted that overreliance on Medicaid serves as a barrier to improving quality of care for people with ADRD. Each state's Medicaid program funds are controlled by the respective state's budget office. State budget offices are usually under a state constitutional requirement for a balanced budget. This leaves funding for state Medicaid vulnerable to political pressure, and people with Alzheimer's and their families are usually not the most politically empowered constituents of the state budget offices.

Vladeck noted that there are ways to improve quality of care without financial incentives. He offered an example from his time as a member of the quality improvement committee of a large nonprofit health care system. The health care system decided to adopt a series of quality recommendations developed by the Institute for Healthcare Improvement (IHI) before Medicare began incentivizing adoption. He said the committee made this decision based on its belief that "good care should not be any more expensive than bad care." Medicare does not provide additional reimbursement to age-friendly hospitals for improving the quality of care for older adult patients. However, that has not prevented those hospitals from implementing those programs. Vladeck posited that health care organizations want to improve care for their patients, and behavioral evidence indicates that they are not motivated primarily by money.

Vladeck suggested that the effective approaches for restructuring the health care system's approach to service delivery should be considered prior to engaging new payment mechanisms. A reworked system needs to accommodate the three main contexts in which people with ADRD receive care and services: hospitals and primary care practices, nursing homes, and home care. Primary care physicians may require incentives to improve initial assessment of patients with possible cognitive impairment. He said this could be accomplished through a combination of training, payment, and professional standards. Many individuals in the later stages of ADRD are best cared for in the second context, nursing homes. However, Vladeck, who served on the committee for a previous Institute of Medicine (IOM) report about quality of care in nursing homes 35 years ago, noted the findings and recommendations of the recent National Academies nursing home consensus study report were "distressingly similar" to those from that 1986 IOM report (IOM, 1986; NASEM, 2022). He added that while the quality issues in nursing homes have remained unchanged, reimbursements per resident are "three to four times" higher than they were 35 years ago. Vladeck said the nursing home industry needs systemic reform before it can be seriously considered for value-based payment models.

Seventy-five percent of people with ADRD receive care in the third context, their home. This is where an overwhelming majority of those patients prefer to reside and receive care. However, he added, there is a shortage of home care workers; a lack of effective quality standards; and no organizational infrastructure with which to manage issues of human resources, payment, incentives, quality, oversight, and customer support. The private home care industry is inadequately regulated. Medicaid pays large amounts of administrative costs to employment agencies that provide home care aides to patients. Vladeck noted that most reimbursed in-home care for people with advanced ADRD is provided by women of color, including many immigrants. Those individuals are underpaid and receive few or no benefits, training, or career opportunities, which is both an equity issue and a quality-of-care issue. He said that improving care for people living with ADRD requires addressing the needs, training, management, and supervision of the home health workforce.

PAYING (ATTENTION TO) UNPAID CAREGIVERS

Emily Largent, Emanuel and Robert Hart Assistant Professor of Medical Ethics and Health Policy at the University of Pennsylvania, began by noting that despite the long history of unpaid caregiving, there is limited published research in the literature about unpaid caregivers, who are frequently family members, for people with ADRD.[3] Family members often manage, finance, and provide care for people with ADRD, who in turn worry about burdening their families. Largent noted two dimensions of inequity that make ADRD more burdensome than other illnesses. ADRD presents greater financial risk and hardship to families than other illnesses. Also, there are considerable disparities within dementia care based on a patient's ability to pay. She added that personal long-term planning frequently cannot compensate for the structural problems within the public insurance systems related to financing ADRD care for older adults.

The overreliance on unpaid caregivers is a national problem, said Largent. In 2021, over 11 million Americans provided unpaid care for people with ADRD, contributing an estimated 16 billion hours valued at $271.6 billion (Alzheimer's Association, 2022). She opined that while efforts have been directed to calculating the cost of ADRD care in terms of the market value of these hours and labeling it as a public health crisis, a similar level of effort has not been directed at developing effective solutions to reduce the pressures placed on caregivers. Family caregivers also play a significant role in long-term care facilities, where they serve as an "invisible workforce" attending to their relatives (Coe and Werner, 2022). This work often includes tasks of feeding, bathing, dressing, grooming, and toileting, as well as care for the mind. Family caregivers make countless care and treatment decisions for the person with ADRD and function as repositories of knowledge about that person's needs and interests, connecting them to their past self. She added that most of the emotional, physical, and economic costs of caregiving for people living with ADRD are borne by women, and particularly women of color. She noted that both paid and unpaid caregiving raises ethical issues around gender, race, ethnicity, and class.

Largent said the COVID-19 pandemic has provided a demonstration of what happens when care is compromised in an already fragile system. Since the onset of the pandemic, caregivers in both community and long-term care settings have experienced negative health outcomes and role strain. Caregivers

---

[3] Largent calculated the number of documents published per year that contain terms *Alzheimer's disease*, *Alzheimer's*, or *Alzheimer* and *caregiver*, as found in the PubMed online database. Similar results were found in Scopus, Web of Science, and in Google texts.

have had increased rates of anxiety and depression. Concurrently, many people living with ADRD have experienced worsening of cognitive and behavioral symptoms and increased falls. There was also a prolonged period during the first year of the pandemic during which families of patients in nursing homes and other long-term care facilities were unable to visit or feed them, leading to weight loss and an attenuation of the family bond. Largent said that the COVID-19 pandemic has revealed the tenuousness of informal caregiving for people with ADRD, even in normal times, and underscores the need for change.

Caregiver role strain and role gain can affect the well-being of both the caregiver and the person living with ADRD (Rapp and Chao, 2000). She explained that *caregiver role strain* refers to difficulty meeting the demands of the caregiver role. *Caregiver role gain* refers to a sense of personal enrichment related to the caregiving role. Increased role strain has been associated with increased risk of abuse and neglect. It is therefore important to mitigate the objective demands of the caregiving role to decrease role strain, as well as to increase role gain by helping caregivers positively frame their interpretation of these demands and their abilities to meet them. She also cautioned against placing an overemphasis on resilience that can put undue pressure on caregivers to persist in an unjust system.

Largent explained that any intervention at the level of the health care system to improve quality of care for people with ADRD should be organized around the dyad of the person with ADRD and their caregiver to maximize the well-being of both parties. She described several key components of that approach. There should be clear documentation in the EHR of the name and contact information for the person with ADRD's caregiver. This would be particularly helpful in recruiting for pragmatic trials specific to patients with ADRD and their caregivers. Best practices should be developed for communication involving the clinician, caregiver, and person with ADRD during clinic visits, including identifying scheduling strategies to allow for adequate appointment duration. Unpaid caregivers should be provided coaching and counseling to equip them with necessary skills, such as skin care and strategies to address common behavioral issues. Additional necessary components that Largent cited include reimbursement for social workers; increased access to respite care; collaborative ADRD care models; and ADRD care navigators, particularly to support care transitions. She added that health care facilities, including hospitals, should revise visitor policies to recognize that caregivers are not typical visitors, they are part of the patient care workforce and often serve as "the extended mind" of a person living with ADRD.

Largent noted that people with ADRD who are un-befriended (those without family, friends, or other unpaid caregivers) are particularly vulnerable to poor care and poor outcomes. She added that people with advanced ADRD that reside in nursing homes who have no visitors usually receive lower quality of care than those with visitors. She emphasized that more research is needed to understand how best to address the unique care needs of these individuals.

DISCUSSION

Addressing Financial Burdens to Caregivers

Richard Frank noted the financial disruptions associated with caregiving for people with ADRD and asked panelists to discuss options for designing more social insurance programs to support caregivers, such as paid family leave policies or provisions in Social Security Administration (SSA) disability insurance. In response, Vladeck said that there have been many such proposals, but they have been superseded by other priorities, such as childcare. Navathe articulated several challenges to Frank's proposal. He began by explaining that payment reform models, such as ACOs and Medicare Advantage, seek to yield improved health outcomes in a manner that is cost neutral for the government and taxpayers. Therefore, a program to support caregivers would likely require finding a different funding source. Second, Navathe cautioned against medicalizing the provision of social services for people at high risk for poor medical outcomes and their families and then evaluating these services based on their cost-effectiveness and their effect on the medical system. He added that those commonly applied evaluation approaches could be problematic for quantifying the effect of social service supports. Navathe noted that success of a caregiver support program might be judged differently depending on whether it was specifically designed for caregivers of people with ADRD or applied more broadly.

Sherry noted that Medicaid HCBS consumer self-direction waivers provide some resources for unpaid family caregivers. There has been increased uptake of this program during the COVID-19 pandemic as people sought to keep family members out of institutions. The limited labor supply of unpaid caregivers is a significant constraint for this program. Many family members cannot provide constant care, particularly as ADRD progresses. Therefore the need remains for mechanisms to support paid caregivers who can supplement unpaid care. She added that existing waiver programs (which vary state by state) could not adequately reimburse family caregivers for constant care, even if they could provide it.

Vladeck noted that if a person with ADRD requires constant care that cannot be provided by an unpaid caregiver, care in a nursing home is less expensive than paying for constant home care. He suggested a possible approach could be an incentive-based payment system that would provide a percentage of the cost of nursing home care to families caring for Medicaid-eligible individuals at home. However, such a proposal would exacerbate the inequities experienced by people with low incomes that are still above the income level for Medicaid eligibility, he added.

Designing a Family Caregiving Support Program

Frank asked the group to discuss the research needs for designing a financial program to support family caregiving for people with ADRD. Navathe suggested one approach could be to conduct demonstration projects in which health plans, clinician groups, or health systems provide funding for caregiver support. Then, test these models rigorously to ensure they are meeting patient and caregiver needs. This would be a longitudinal, multi-year project. Navathe described several requirements for this approach, including identifying the critical elements of caregiving, determining how those critical elements connect with the medical enterprise care model, testing financing approaches for facilitating payments to caregivers, and developing assessment mechanisms for valuation and impact. Sherry added that there is considerable heterogeneity in the goals and preferences of patients and their families, which may change over the trajectory of disease. She said that one starting point for researchers may be to identify universal goals for both patients and caregivers, and then investigate at what point in the trajectory of ADRD the goals fail to align. An example research question could be, what key antecedents lead to an inability to remain at home? Sherry listed several possible factors that could contribute to the divergence of goals for people with ADRD and their caregivers. Those included behavioral or psychological symptoms, burnout, depression, labor supply, and housing. She noted that there is a substantial volume of research about those factors published in the literature. She suggested examining the existing evidence for opportunities to integrate those findings and identify potential solutions that can inform actionable policy recommendations.

Institutionalization and De-institutionalization Challenges

Hollmann and Vladeck briefly discussed the roles of institutionalization and deinstitutionalization in care models for patients with ADRD. Hollmann suggested modeling the effects of transferring financing from institutional care to home care for people with ADRD. He added that any modeling should incorporate characteristics of the desired conditions, such as accounting for better wages for nursing home staff, instead of current conditions.

Vladeck recounted the example of deinstitutionalization at New York's Willowbrook facility. The children with developmental disabilities who were residents at Willowbrook and were deinstitutionalized are now adults with developmental disabilities that are also experiencing a range of medical problems as they age, including early-onset dementia. Those individuals frequently cannot be cared for adequately in community facilities so they become residents in nursing homes. This adds to the multidimensional diversity and diversity of needs of people with ADRD residing in nursing homes. He added that adapting to the diversity in the population of people with ADRD and the evolution of that diversity over time will add complexity to the issue of providing adequate and equitable ADRD treatment.

Scaling

Frank noted that several effective care models for people with ADRD described by speakers were examples of "expensive boutique operations," and asked the group to discuss the essential components of those expensive small models that could be scaled up to develop a workable and effective large-scale model. Vladeck suggested developing institutional models and creating regionally based centers that could translate the lessons from smaller-scale programs into operational practices and lobby for the adjustments in payment policy needed to make these models more widely available. Sherry added that regional collaborative centers could offer the opportunity to marshal other types of resources and build from the community up, bringing together components that are outside the medical system but still critical to the success of the care models.

Drawing on his prior work in behavioral economics and science, Navathe noted that the decrease in effect size that is observed when efforts are made to generalize a boutique model is a common and challenging problem. He noted that in behavioral science this is referred to as the voltage effect.[4] Innovation should take place in smaller settings because the unique nature and intensity of the needs of people with ADRD are difficult to generalize. This makes large-scale efforts at innovation likely to fail. However, while small-scale innovation is needed to generate the best care models, there should be a deliberate effort to identify the common elements across successful models. He noted that support for caregivers is an advantageous feature to add to a care model because it contributes to a patient-centered approach and is scalable. He also noted that it could be challenging to incorporate that component because caregiver support is not a single service.

Sherry added that several elements of evidence-based ADRD care models are similar to those for individuals with other complex medical conditions and long-term care needs. She suggested identifying common elements in the two types of models as well as identifying modifications needed to address the

---

[4] See https://www.penguinrandomhouse.com/books/672117/the-voltage-effect-by-john-a-list/ (accessed July 16, 2022).

distinctive needs of people living with ADRD. She said that this approach may facilitate scaling, because a large health care delivery organization may be more willing to invest in a new care model if it is designed to serve a broader patient population.

Resources for Information About Quality

Fulmer recommended four resources that represent opportunities to enhance the evidence base regarding quality of care for people living with ADRD and support for their caregivers:

- The Family Caregiver Alliance,[5]
- HRSA's Geriatrics Workforce Enhancement Program,[6]
- The Veterans Administration,[7] and
- The Administration for Community Living.[8]

---

[5] See https://www.caregiver.org (accessed July 16, 2022).

[6] See https://www.americangeriatrics.org/programs/gwep-coordinating-center (accessed July 16, 2022).

[7] See https://www.caregiver.va.gov/index.asp (accessed July 16, 2022).

[8] See https://acl.gov (accessed July 16, 2022).

5

Evidence on the Effect of Existing Models and Research and Innovation to Address Gaps in Data and Evidence

In this session, panelists discussed innovative programs for providing and funding care for people with Alzheimer's disease and related dementias (ADRD).

EXISTING MODELS FOR FUNDING CARE FOR PEOPLE WITH ADRD

Julie Robison, professor of medicine, Center on Aging at the University of Connecticut School of Medicine, described two existing models of funding care for people with ADRD, Money Follows the Person (MFP) and Care of Persons with Dementia in their Environments (COPE). She began with an explanation of the CMS project Money Follows the Person (MFP). MFP aims to provide choice to individuals with ADRD regarding where to live and receive services by strengthening Medicaid's ability to support people who want to transition out of institutions such as nursing homes or skilled nursing facilities.[1] This is done by eliminating barriers at the state level that restrict the use of Medicaid funds and strengthening the ability of Medicaid programs to provide home- and community-based services (HCBS) to these individuals. In 2008, CMS undertook an MFP demonstration that included 46 states, the District of Columbia, as well as an initiative for Native Americans. She said

---

[1] See https://www.medicaid.gov/medicaid/long-term-services-supports/money-follows-person/index.html (accessed June 10, 2022).

that by 2020, over 107,000 people in the MFP demonstration projects had transitioned to community living.

MFP is a voluntary program open to people of all ages and disabilities who are eligible for Medicaid, have been in an institution for at least 90 days, and would like to transition to receiving care and supports at home. This includes people with ADRD and other neurodegenerative conditions. The MFP transition planning process is initiated when a patient, their family, or a nursing home staff member submits a referral for transition. At that point a transition team is assembled. This team includes the patient, family members, nursing home staff, regional transition coordinators, community program care managers, housing coordinators, and others, depending on the individual's unique needs. The goal of the transition team is developing and executing a community-based, person-centered long-term service and support (LTSS) plan to coordinate the person's care in the community. In the Connecticut MFP program, there have been over 7,000 transitions since 2009. That includes people ages 1 to 104 years with 45 percent older than 65 and 40 percent under 65 with physical disabilities. Thirteen percent of people that transitioned to home in the Connecticut program had a specific ADRD diagnosis. Twenty-five percent of the people that transitioned home identified as not White and 11 percent identified as Hispanic.

Robison studied individuals in the Connecticut MFP program for two years following their transition and found positive outcomes, which are mirrored in the national evaluation data from Mathematica (Kellett et al., 2021; Mathematica, 2017; Robison et al., 2015).[2] Individuals reported improved quality of life and life satisfaction following the transition. This improvement was sustained for the entire two-year follow-up period. Only 10 to12 percent of people returned to an institution in the first year. Family caregivers reported lower levels of burden than are typically observed. Robison attributed this to support in the form of a paid care plan that includes supports that supplement the caregiver's work (Robison et al., 2021).

Robison noted several areas for improvement. Individuals had a slightly increased rate of falls and more frequent emergency department (ED) and hospital visits following transition to home (Marrero et al., 2019). She also identified systemic factors that have limited success of MFP demonstrations, including the severe HCBS workforce shortage; variation in MFP programs across states, some of which are very small and siloed; the slow pace of transition from facility to home, which can take years in some cases; and the need for more proactive identification of eligible individuals (Robison et al., 2020).

---

[2] See https://www.mathematica.org/projects/research-and-evaluation-of-the-money-follows-the-person-mfp-demonstration-grants (accessed June 10, 2022).

She added that despite these limitations, MFP has had many success stories in Connecticut.[3]

Robison next explained the COPE program. COPE is designed to address the particular needs of the dyad of the person living with ADRD and their caregiver. COPE is driven by occupational therapists (OTs), who develop action plans with the caregiver and complete up to 10 home visits over the course of 16 weeks.[4] The program also includes a home visit from a nurse practitioner who assesses dehydration, pain, and other symptoms and takes biological samples for lab tests. The nurse practitioner then conducts a follow-up call with the caregiver to review the results of the lab tests and coordinate communication of those results with the patient's primary care physician. COPE was found to be efficacious in a randomized controlled trial with community-based participants (Gitlin et al., 2010).

Robison's colleague at the University of Connecticut tested the program in the COPE CT Translational Study. This study tested the effectiveness and implementation of COPE in a real-world setting, using an existing Medicaid-funded HCBS program for older adults (Fortinsky et al., 2020). Prior to COPE, the existing HCBS program offered no services to help family caregivers improve their ADRD management skills, though approximately one third of the 16,000 clients had ADRD. Researchers observed many positive outcomes for caregivers and people living with ADRD, as well as reduced system costs (Fortinsky et al., 2020; Kellett et al., 2022; Pizzi et al., 2022). Caregivers reported substantial improvement in their ability to manage the target problem areas, with 96 percent of respondents reporting reduction or resolution of these particular target problems at the end of the intervention.

Robison noted that in order to scale up COPE, Medicare and Medicaid coverage will need to be streamlined. She also suggested that while Medicare and Medicaid currently reimburse OT and registered nurse (RN) services, a bundled payment model, such as those currently used in Medicare Advantage or ACOs, may be needed to support ancillary components, such as training, materials, and ongoing coaching. Scalability also depends on development of a network of trained OT/RN COPE providers and referral mechanisms. She added that COPE program materials need to be translated for people that do not speak English.

---

[3] See https://health.uconn.edu/aging/research-reports/ (accessed June 14, 2022). Each quarterly report concludes with the story of an individual MFP client.

[4] See https://drexel.edu/cnhp/research/centers/agewell/Research-Studies/COPE/ (accessed June 14, 2022).

PACE: PROGRAM OF ALL-INCLUSIVE CARE FOR THE ELDERLY

Jennie Chin Hansen, board member of SCAN Health Plan and former chief executive officer of the American Geriatrics Society, began by discussing the Program of All-Inclusive Care for the Elderly (PACE). She explained that PACE is an integrated system for older adults who are frail. The program uses a capitated payment model. It is a community-based, coordinated care program that provides a full range of medical and non-medical services. Hansen led the PACE program in San Francisco for 25 years.[5] PACE serves individuals residing within its service areas who are age 55 or older who are certified as needing nursing home care but who are still able to live safely in the community with support from PACE services. PACE clients have functional losses and complex health issues, with an average of 5.8 chronic comorbidities; 46 percent have ADRD. She noted that the PACE client population resembles that of nursing homes, with an average age in the late seventies to early eighties.

Individual PACE centers are small in scale, serving approximately 200 people. An important component of PACE is that the program engages an interdisciplinary team rather than individual case managers to manage care. The team includes OTs, physical therapists, recreational therapists, primary care providers, RNs, social workers, dietitians, home care coordinators, personal care attendants, and drivers. The team focuses on prevention at multiple levels and engages in a continuous process of assessment, treatment planning, service provision, and monitoring. PACE has strong core competencies that support its broader use, said Hansen. It is provider based, provider directed, and provider managed, with tightly controlled systems of care management and utilization. PACE has consistently demonstrated several positive quality indicators, including good care outcomes, high enrollee and caregiver satisfaction, and low rates of disenrollment (CMS, 2018). PACE also proved effective at mitigating COVID-19 transmission during the pandemic, with rates of infection and death approximately two-thirds lower than in skilled nursing facilities.

PACE financing is capitated and pooled, integrating payments from Medicare, Medicaid, and private payers, said Hansen. Ninety percent of enrollees are eligible for both Medicaid and Medicare, with the Medicare capitation rate adjusted for the frailty of the enrollees. Home care is covered, as are services such as audiology, dentistry, podiatry, and other supports, such as air conditioning. She noted that PACE now has 144 participating providers with close to 300 sites in 30 states. She said an upcoming report from the Bipartisan Policy Center will discuss mechanisms for its expansion.

---

[5] See https://www.npaonline.org (accessed June 15, 2022).

Hansen next discussed a collaboration among the American College of Emergency Physicians, the Society for Academic Emergency Medicine, the American Geriatrics Society, and the Emergency Nurses Association to develop accredited geriatric emergency departments (GEDs).[6] There are currently approximately 275 GEDs around the United States, and the Veterans Administration (VA) is committed to providing GEDs in every VA hospital emergency department (Kennedy et al., 2022).[7] In San Francisco, the University of California–San Francisco, Kaiser Health in San Francisco, the Zuckerberg General Hospital and Trauma Center, and the Dolby Family Foundation have supported research to identify validated screening tools that can be appropriately used in EDs. The particular lens of ADRD was and continues to be an essential component and research priority for GED program development, said Hansen. She noted that the GED Collaborative, with support from AARP will be producing videos to help GED (and all ED) staff recognize delirium and dementia. Additionally, publications addressing communication, care transitions, and best practices will be published this year.

CARE MODELS FOR OLDER PEOPLE AND PEOPLE WITH ADRD: WORLD HEALTH ORGANIZATION VISION AND CURRENT KNOWLEDGE

Hyobum Jang, technical officer in the Ageing and Health Unit of the World Health Organization (WHO) discussed an international perspective on efforts to improve quality of care and supports for people with ADRD and their caregivers. He began by noting three important reports that have been released in the last decade. The *World Report on Aging and Health* included a focus on the concept of healthy aging, which inspired the United Nations (UN) Decade of Healthy Aging 2021–2030[8] (WHO, 2015). The *Global Action Plan on the Public Health Response to Dementia* focuses on the public health response to dementia, which has been identified as a priority public health issue (WHO, 2017). These reports have led to a convergence of life-course and disease-specific approaches to providing care for people with ADRD and supporting their caregivers, said Jang.

He explained that the UN Decade of Healthy Aging includes four action areas: addressing ageism; developing age-friendly communities; delivering inte-

---

[6] See https://gedcollaborative.com (accessed July 20, 2022).
[7] See https://www.va.gov/opa/pressrel/pressrelease.cfm?id=5712 (accessed July 20, 2022).
[8] See https://www.who.int/initiatives/decade-of-healthy-ageing (accessed July 20, 2022).

grated care responsive to the needs of older people; and providing long-term care for those who need it, which overlaps with ADRD care. The two action areas related to health care are being addressed by WHO. This is being done in part through WHO's Integrated Care for Older People (ICOPE), which seeks to transform health and social care services and systems at multiple levels (WHO, 2022). The WHO vision for long-term care systems includes the provision of services that are people centered, empower older people and caregivers, and provide a continuum of integrated and coordinated care, while responding to the unique health and social care needs and goals of older people. The ICOPE vision also emphasizes the need to address the social determinants of health.

Jang explained that the WHO care model for ADRD is similar to these healthy aging models in its emphasis on a multidisciplinary collaborative approach and active cooperation between paid and unpaid caregivers (WHO, 2017). Proposed actions in the model include embedding a pathway of efficient, coordinated, and person-centered care for people with ADRD into health and social systems and shifting the locus of care from hospitals to multidisciplinary community-based care settings. Multidisciplinary care models for ADRD are effective when integrated within primary care, said Jang, citing a systematic review of ten trials examining a variety of care models (WHO, 2021). He added that primary care physician (PCP)-led care also decreased hospital costs and improved caregiver mental health.

Jang said a WHO study of long-term care (LTC) financing yielded many lessons (Barber et al., 2021). Researchers found that public investments in formal LTC systems are particularly important because of the aging population, reduction in family caregivers, and the difficulty of planning for LTC on an individual level. The study also found that while a separate funding stream for LTC may be helpful, it may also complicate coordination across health care and social care sectors. Another finding of note was that making cost control the primary objective or setting overly stringent eligibility criteria can lead to unmet needs.

Jang discussed three different examples from Qatar, Australia, and Korea to illustrate some of the ways different countries were addressing the care needs of older people. He began with an example from Qatar, a small country with high income. The country recently initiated a national system of care for older people that includes coordinated social and health care services in the home setting, specialized teams focused on restoring patients' functional independence in the long-term inpatient setting, specialized care centers for older people that focus on a person-centered approach, and community-based residential care services to help patients transition from acute care to the home (WHO, 2021). The strength of this program is the presence of a dedicated geriatric unit in the main health center that collaborates with local service centers to provide integrated care for older people. In addition, under its

National Mental Health Strategy, Qatar is transitioning from hospital-based toward community-based mental health services (Sharkey, 2017).[9]

Jang next discussed an example from Australia. The state of New South Wales, Australia, operates a program in Western Sydney for older people with chronic and complex health needs. The model is community based, patient focused, and coordinated between home and hospital (McNab and Gillespie, 2015).[10] A general practice liaison nurse visits the home, identifies needs, and coordinates care among providers, with patients and caregivers actively participating in care planning and management. Care is delivered in the most appropriate settings by multidisciplinary teams. Although positive outcomes have been observed, this program is new and is funded from multiple sources that do not cover all physician costs, making implementation challenging, noted Jang. Australia also has a countrywide transition care program that provides 12 to 18 weeks of services to older people in their homes following a hospital stay, with the goal of improving their independence and transitioning them to community living, said Jang (WHO, 2021).

Jang next discussed an example from South Korea. South Korea provides universal long-term care insurance (LTCI), managed by its single-payer national health insurance system. People over 65 or with specific geriatric diseases, including ADRD, are eligible for LTCI (Barber et al., 2021). In 2018, 8.4 percent of people over 65 received services covered by LTCI. In 2019, 54.5 percent of LTCI expenditures were for home-based care, including visiting nursing, bathing, day and night care, and short-term care. He noted that LTCI only covers care provided by formal paid providers. Among people who received LTCI, 89 percent received some support from family members. This has contributed to high rates of caregiver burden, mostly among female relatives, said Jang, who also noted a lack of coordination between the health and social care systems.

Jang noted that the need for integrated care for older people and people with ADRD, particularly long-term care for people with ADRD, has gained attention in the United States and globally. Many current models focus on care coordination, continuum of care, and integration at both the system level and among providers. Worldwide, the growing burden for informal caregivers and the need to provide better supports remains a challenge. He said that more concrete evidence is needed to enable countries, including lower- and middle-income economies, to adapt appropriate care models for their specific contexts.

---

[9] See https://www.moph.gov.qa/english/strategies/Supporting-Strategies-and-Frameworks/SummaryNationalMentalHealthFramework2019-2022/Pages/default.aspx (accessed July 20, 2022).

[10] Case study is from an upcoming WHO, 2022, report, *A Service Package of Long-Term Care Interventions*.

ALTERNATIVE PAYMENT MODELS FOR ADRD CARE

Peter Hollmann, chief medical officer of Brown Medicine and board chair of the American Geriatrics Society, discussed alternative payment mechanisms for ADRD care. He explained that it is possible to incentivize changes in care delivery systems. Medicare, Medicare Advantage, and many commercial insurance plans use a variety of rewards and penalties to reduce cost and increase quality of care. Although incentives are insufficient on their own, they can create a shift in mindset, he added. That change of mindset incentivized implementation of programs like the Hospital Elder Life Program (HELP), Care of Vulnerable Elders (COVE), the Geriatric ED, and palliative care. Alternative payment mechanisms were developed to prioritize value over volume and to emphasize budgetary accountability in the health care system. He noted that these alternative mechanisms require flexibility to enable providers to direct their spending to attain specific goals. Medicare Advantage is one of the earliest examples of alternative payment mechanisms. He opined that the separation between Medicare Advantage and general Medicare may create challenges for scaling models and ideas across both programs.

He noted that while often criticized, the fee-for-service payment model is flexible and widely available. He explained that Current Procedural Terminology (CPT) codes used in fee-for-service models offer an opportunity to create new service descriptions in response to coverage changes. Hollmann served on a panel that created new CPT codes, including Transitional Care Management and Chronic Care Management, to facilitate CMS payment for services offered within medical homes. Use of both codes was associated with improvements in cost and quality by independent reviewers (Bindman and Cox, 2018; Schurrer et al., 2017). Services provided under these codes are reimbursable by Medicare whether they are performed by licensed medical professionals or unlicensed clinical staff when they are supervised by a physician, advanced practice registered nurse (APRN), or physician assistant (PA). However, those codes do not include services provided by community-based organizations. This complicates analyses to determine whether the service might lead to long-term savings. He said that in 2024 additional CPT codes will be released that address informal caregiving, include caregiver training provided by OTs or PTs to enhance patient functional performance, caregiver behavior management training, and telemedicine.[11]

Alternative payment mechanisms (APMs) specific to patients with ADRD have been proposed, and their cost-effectiveness is well supported in the literature (Boustani et al., 2019; Haggerty et al., 2020). This research is critical

---

[11] See https://www.ama-assn.org/amaone/cpt-current-procedural-terminology (accessed July 20, 2022).

EXISTING MODELS AND RESEARCH

because it can encourage health care plans to implement disease-specific CPT programs even in the absence of a disease-specific APM, he added. Disease-specific APMs have encountered several challenges. There are complex design issues, including challenges determining which physicians or organizations get paid for which services, and there can be difficulties in scaling and replication. Hollmann noted that many have encountered delays during consideration by the Physician-Focused Payment Model Technical Advisory Committee (PTAC).[12] The Medicare Payment Advisory Commission (MedPAC)[13] has recommended ceasing the addition of new APMs.

Hollmann encouraged implementation of existing APMs and incentive programs. He noted one example, the Medicare Shared Savings Program,[14] which uses a risk-adjusted budget but does not reimburse care and services provided by non-licensed staff, such as informal caregivers. Another example is Primary Care First,[15] which provides infrastructure support, a telehealth waiver, and risk adjustment for the whole practice. It does not include additional reimbursement for care for patients with ADRD. He noted that it makes Primary Care First unlikely to change the behavior of physicians who see a small number of patients with ADRD. Another APM, Comprehensive Primary Care Plus (CPC Plus), does include additional reimbursement for providing care for people with ADRD. None of these programs include support infrastructure for community services. He noted that an obvious approach to avoiding ADRD quality-of-care issues associated with care transitions is to avoid hospitalization. While quality primary care for people with ADRD can reduce the need for hospitalization, supports from promising programs, such as Independence at Home and Hospital at Home, could also be beneficial.

DISCUSSION

How the Models Support Care Transitions Across Settings

Inouye asked the speakers to discuss how the various models addressed care transitions for people with ADRD. Robison explained that MFP is focused on improving the quality of care during transitions. Reimbursement funds that would have been spent on care in a nursing home are made available for

---

[12] See https://aspe.hhs.gov/collaborations-committees-advisory-groups/ptac (accessed July 22, 2022).

[13] See https://www.medpac.gov (accessed July 22, 2022).

[14] See https://www.cms.gov/Medicare/Medicare-Fee-for-Service-Payment/sharedsavingsprogram/about (accessed July 22, 2022).

[15] See https://innovation.cms.gov/innovation-models/primary-care-first-model-options (accessed July 22, 2022).

the person when they return to the community. As a result, states also get a larger federal match on their Medicaid funds. All of the resources provided in MFP are focused on establishing a care plan to support the person when they reenter the community. The program requires participants to transition into an existing community-based program, such as the Connecticut Home Care Program for Elders.[16] The community-based program assigns a case manager who contacts the person monthly, visits semiannually, and is involved during subsequent care transitions and hospitalizations. She explained that COPE focuses on educating caregivers, improving caregivers' resources, and achieving better coordination between the caregiver and PCP. Integration of COPE into a community-based program provides additional services to people living with ADRD.

Robison noted that these programs are not perfect. Robison observed increased rehospitalizations, ED visits, and falls among individuals in MFP despite deliberate efforts to integrate health care needs with community-based services. Inouye suggested that information technology and communications strategies might help address those challenges. Robison noted that American Rescue Plan Act funds are being directed for supporting value-based payments to HCBS providers to enable them to access data within the Connecticut Heath Information Exchange (HIE).[17,18] Robison said this should enable development of incentives, targeting, and risk identification to prevent care transitions due to avoidable hospitalizations. Primary care providers, nursing homes, and hospitals are already part of Connecticut's HIE, and Robison suggested that integrating HCBS into this system is a promising reform.

Hansen added that the goal with care and support for people living with ADRD is to help them remain in their best and most stable functional state and ensure they encounter as few challenges as possible in the course of their daily lives. This requires preparation, anticipation, and then mitigation when something goes awry. Hansen noted that the public health concept of primary, secondary, and tertiary forms of prevention applies to care transitions. She offered an example of this approach, helping the caregiver anticipate clinical and behavioral changes and mitigate their effects can reduce avoidable ED visits and hospital stays. Hansen suggested that data can be used to help guide the family through care transitions for a person with ADRD, ensuring that the necessary equipment, medication, and care are ready before the person comes

---

[16] See https://portal.ct.gov/DSS/Health-And-Home-Care/Connecticut-Home-Care-Program-for-Elders/Connecticut-Home-Care-Program-for-Elders-CHCPE (accessed July 22, 2022).

[17] See https://www.whitehouse.gov/american-rescue-plan/ (accessed July 22, 2022).

[18] See https://conniect.org (accessed July 22, 2022).

home from the hospital. She emphasized that preparation, anticipation, and mitigation can help promote stability for patients, caregivers, and clinicians.

Jang noted that while none of the international models are perfect in their approach to care transitions, one consistently important feature is care coordination. Care coordination enables the person with ADRD to be referred to appropriate health and social services without requiring the family to identify these services themselves. Another important feature is the provision of support for caregivers in home and community settings, including training, education, and respite care. A third feature is continuous monitoring and assessment. He said the care coordinator and care provider should be continuously involved in monitoring and assessing the person's changing care needs to enable smooth transitions.

Inouye noted that in several Asian countries where the populations are aging extremely rapidly, the need for caregivers has reached urgent levels. She added that this has led to development of some innovative models, such as a Japanese program that trains young volunteers to learn about care of older adults. Jang said there are growing efforts to train community members, both younger and older people, to act as caregivers. There are also experimental joint living facilities where older people can live together and support one another, similar to aging-in-place communities, though these are limited to people who can function relatively independently, he noted.

Hollmann explained that hospital readmissions are expensive and are also a common quality measure, which has made them a focus of many quality improvement programs. People with ADRD are among those most likely to be readmitted, which has encouraged changes to their care, including the establishment of home visit programs. Hollmann is working to strengthen the home visit program in Rhode Island, particularly for people recently discharged from the hospital. Rhode Island has also enhanced notifications through HIEs. He suggested a national HIE would be beneficial to improve visibility and access to information about care transitions. He added that published research has demonstrated that this is important for cost and quality.

How the Models Match Patients' Goals and Priorities to the Care They Receive

Inouye next asked the group to discuss how current programs and payment policies match the goals and priorities of the patient with ADRD to the care they receive. Hollmann began by explaining that while current PCP-managed programs may not explicitly address patients' goals, there are certain aspects that promote matching care to patient goals. The relationship with the primary care clinician is an important feature, as are the care management staff, who are attuned to supporting people with ADRD to express their goals. Under Primary Care First, advanced care planning is a quality measure that must be raised during the annual wellness visit, said Hollmann. Additionally, patient surveys ask about patients' overall perception of care and whether they felt that care included shared decision making.[19] Hollmann suggested that patient surveys provided when patients leave the hospital should include a question that asks, "Is the care you are receiving consistent with your expectations and goals?" He noted that individuals may prefer less expensive care options, such as avoiding hospital stays or establishing advance directives.

Robison said that ascertaining the patient's goals is a strength of both MFP and COPE. COPE works with the dyad, gaining input on goals from both the person with ADRD and the caregiver. MFP is voluntary, with eligibility predicated on the person's desire to transition to the community, and the care plan is developed in accordance with their goals. The Consumer Assessment of Healthcare Providers and Systems (CAHPS) survey used for HCBS in Connecticut addresses this specifically. She noted that the survey includes questions such as, "Does your care plan include the things that are important to you?" and "Does your caregiver know the things that are important to you?" Robison noted that patients' goals are context dependent. A person's health care goals will differ from their daily living goals. These different goals will require different types of services. Moreover, these goals are prioritized differently across individual patients, said Robison, highlighting the importance of the What Matters Movement.

How the Models Address Health Care Disparities in Underrepresented Groups

Inouye next asked the group to discuss how the models discussed can address health care disparities experienced by people from historically underrepresented communities. Hansen explained that the original PACE program was started in a historically marginalized community. The first efforts at replication of the PACE program were predominantly in communities that have historically been marginalized and made vulnerable. When she started the replications, many Black people did not use nursing homes, either because they were not available or because they did not feel comfortable. She added that 34 years later, PACE programs serving these same populations in South Carolina and around the country are robust.

Jang said that WHO is examining equity-related issues in caregiving. He

---

[19] See https://www.cms.gov/Medicare/Quality-Initiatives-Patient-Assessment-Instruments/HospitalQualityInits/HospitalHCAHPS (accessed July 22, 2022).

noted that in countries where formal home caregiving is not provided, that role is filled by family members, mostly women, who frequently experience job loss and increasing mental and physical stress, without support or respite. He also highlighted the existence of disparities between individual households, with some able to hire informal caregivers. However, this informal economy contributes to additional disparities, with paid informal caregivers largely being people from historically marginalized communities or immigrants. Advocating for these caregivers is one goal of the UN Decade of Healthy Aging,[20] he added. Inouye underscored the need to address the exacerbation of inequities and often severe financial problems that result from overreliance on informal caregivers, who are often women.

How the Models Address Health Outcomes and Care Processes

Inouye then asked the group to describe how the models they discussed address health outcomes and care processes for people with ADRD, such as fall prevention, restraint use, management of mentation, and delirium prevention, as well as the frequent complications of hospitalization, severe illness, and multi-morbidities. Hansen began by explaining that PACE programs have close relationships and good communication with their contracted hospitals. This enables PACE providers to anticipate when a member will be discharged and to gain specific information regarding their health and behavior. This reflects a structural process: development of a working relationship that enables person-centric knowledge to be communicated effectively in both directions. The PACE team monitors patients while they are in nursing homes, including regular site visits. She noted that being familiar with the person and their range of normal behaviors can help another party care for them safely and appropriately. In addition, individual patients are discussed at daily team meetings and weekly formal meetings. These meetings provide teaching opportunities and continuing education on delirium prevention and other topics.

Hollmann said that most health care organizations have an inherent interest in implementing safety measures, as unsafe conditions usually increase cost, length-of-stay, and the likelihood of needing post-acute care. He also cautioned against creating excessive measurement burdens for the primary care setting. He added that this risks diverting provider focus away from more important issues or causing unintended problems, similar to when efforts to avert falls in hospitals lead to patient immobility. He suggested that the patient experience of care, with a goal of ensuring that care goals are consistent with both the patient's and the caregiver's needs, could be the most important element to measure.

---

[20] See https://www.who.int/initiatives/decade-of-healthy-ageing (accessed September 28, 2022).

Robison explained that COPE's combination of an OT and nurse, combined with its individualized approach, supports patient safety. The OT becomes knowledgeable about the individual person with ADRD, which enables them to provide more specific recommendations for exercises. The nurse practitioner can detect undiagnosed conditions through lab tests and share that information with the primary care provider. However, COPE is a one-time program that does not continue through the duration of the disease, while the person with ADRD continues to change over time. She suggested this creates an opportunity to explore changes to the program to support longitudinal follow-up.

6

Creating Change

Faith Mitchell introduced the final workshop session as an examination of promising new opportunities for change in care for people with ADRD. Speakers addressed the individual, the community, and health care settings, as well as workforce challenges and modifications of payment models. Concerns specific to ADRD care were integrated with important insights about behavior and systems change, with a focus on the patient's perspective.

CHANGING BEHAVIORS TO SUPPORT BRAIN HEALTH

Sarah Lenz Lock, senior vice president for policy and brain health in the AARP Policy, Research, and International Affairs Department and executive director of the Global Council on Brain Health, explained that up to 40 percent of dementias could be prevented by modifiable lifestyle factors (Livingston, 2020). These interventions can delay onset of dementia, reduce risk, and improve the quality of life for people living with ADRD. Lenz Lock urged researchers to consider managing dementia as a chronic disease in which it is possible to improve quality of life. She added that frequently there is a disconnect between health care providers and individuals when it comes to awareness of these modifiable lifestyle factors. Recent AARP surveys found that a substantial majority of health care providers know that regular exercise, social interactions, healthy diet, adequate sleep, stress management, and mental stimulation can improve the quality of life of people living with dementia, and a substantial majority of adults were willing to adopt these behaviors if they understood they were beneficial to their brain health. However, she opined that the benefits of those modifiable lifestyle factors to brain health are not adequately disseminated to patients and are frequently overlooked by research efforts directed at improving quality of care for people with ADRD.

Lenz Lock suggested that the stigma associated with ADRD, which may cause discomfort among health care providers, may contribute to less forthright conversations when discussing an ADRD diagnosis with a patient. Young providers may not understand how their older patients feel or their priorities. Research conducted by AARP revealed that the two groups differ substantially in their feelings about an ADRD diagnosis. The organization surveyed adults age 40 and older as well as health care providers about their feelings about a dementia diagnosis. Nineteen percent of respondents from the adults age 40 and older group agreed with the statement, "If I had dementia, I would be ashamed or embarrassed" (AARP, 2021). However, 69 percent of health care providers agreed with a similar statement, "If my patient had dementia, they would be ashamed or embarrassed" (AARP, 2021). In the same survey, 7 percent of respondents age 40 and older agreed with the statement, "If I had dementia, I would give up on life" (AARP, 2021). Thirty-two percent of health care providers agreed with the statement, "If my patient had dementia, they would give up on life" (AARP, 2021). She noted that there is a need for many health care providers to overcome their reluctance to talk about dementia and treat it as a manageable chronic disease.

Lenz Lock cited a recent report on behavior change by the Global Council on Brain Health (GCBH)[1] and suggested that some improvements in quality of care can be made within the health care system in the absence of payment reform. The GCBH report makes recommendations for individuals, communities (health care providers, employers, advocates, nonprofits, etc.), and policy makers to support brain health. She suggested that change will be needed at all levels of the health care system. The report includes specific strategies for individuals to engage in to support brain health.[2] She suggested that the most important recommendation that the report makes for communities is to set goals to change behavior in order to improve brain health, which could reduce the stigma associated with ADRD diagnosis.

---

[1] See https://www.aarp.org/health/brain-health/global-council-on-brain-health/behavior-change/ (accessed on June 17, 2022).

[2] See https://www.aarp.org/content/dam/aarp/health/brain_health/2022-03/gcbh-behavior-change-infographic-english.doi.10.26419-2Fpia.00106.002.pdf (accessed on July 28, 2022).

CHANGING CARE TO ADDRESS
THE NEEDS OF PEOPLE LIVING WITH DEMENTIA

Leslie Pelton, vice president, Institute for Healthcare Improvement, began by explaining that determining how to attain reliable, sustainable delivery of evidence-based care that serves the needs of people living with ADRD is essential. The 4 Ms (what *m*atters, *m*edication, *m*entation, and *m*obility) framework represents a set of evidence-based core elements of care for older adults that also represent the core health issues for people living with ADRD (Figure 6-1) (Mate et al., 2021). Adherence to the 4 Ms framework supports patient safety, particularly for patients with ADRD. The framework also simplifies care for people with ADRD for health care providers.

Pelton explained that inclusion of mentation in the 4 Ms supports normalizing the discussion of brain health, with the goal of this discussion

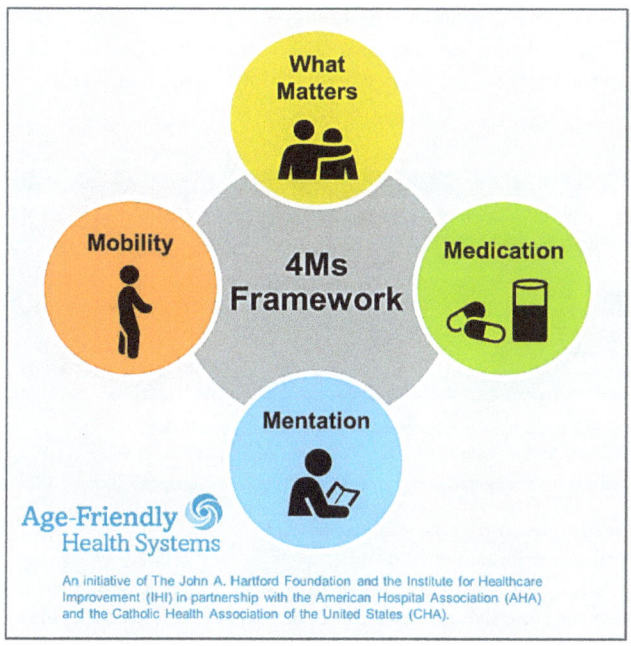

FIGURE 6-1 The 4 Ms framework.
Source: Presented by Leslie Pelton on May 24, 2022 at the workshop Mechanisms for Organizational Behavior Change to Address the Needs of People Living with Alzheimer's Disease and Related Dementias. For related work, this graphic may be used in its entirety without requesting permission. Graphic files and guidance at ihi.org/AgeFriendly. Accessed via ihi.org/AgeFriendly. (Mate et al., 2021).

becoming as normal as a conversation about the health of any other organ and destigmatizing this discussion for health care providers. The "what matters" component, which includes health care providers asking patients and their caregivers, "What matters to you?" helps people with ADRD and their caregivers identify and communicate their goals and priorities. This facilitates organization of care around those answers.[3] There are effective ways to assess whether evidence-based care is being practiced, said Pelton, including measures of access, process, and outcome (Fulmer et al., 2022).[4]

Pelton explained that how the 4 Ms should be practiced in each system where people with ADRD receive care is unknown. This will vary depending on the culture, lived experiences, and technologies available to each individual care team. She added that the combination of firm expectations for use of the 4 Ms as a framework with outcome measures, while also allowing each care team to adapt the framework to their system, can lead to sustainable change (Figure 6-2). The Model for Improvement is a tool for helping health care teams adapt the 4 Ms framework to their particular environments (Langley et al., 2009). The combination of a high level of autonomy and tools to learn and build at the local level supports a more positive experience for the health care team (Perlo et al., 2017).

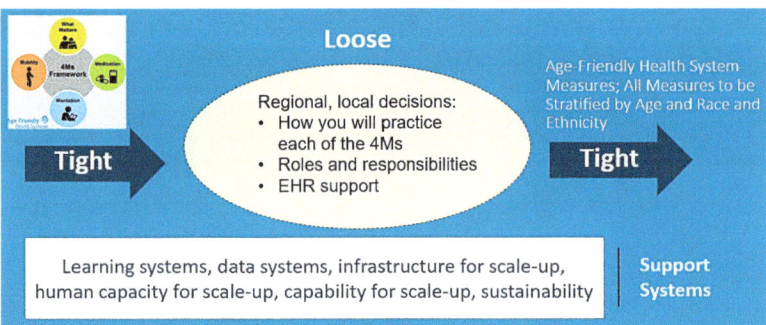

FIGURE 6-2 Implementing the 4 Ms framework.
NOTE: EHR = electronic health record.
SOURCE: Adapted from Barker, P. M., A. Reid, M. W. Schall. A framework for scaling up health interventions: Lessons from large-scale improvement initiatives in Africa. *Implementation Science*. 2016 Jan;11(1):12. Presented by Leslie Pelton on May 24, 2022 at the workshop Mechanisms for Organizational Behavior Change to Address the Needs of People Living with Alzheimer's Disease and Related Dementias. Source of data: Barker et al., 2016.

---

[3] See https://theconversationproject.org/wp-content/uploads/2020/12/Conversation StarterGuide.pdf (accessed June 17, 2022).

[4] See http://www.ihi.org/Engage/Initiatives/Age-Friendly-Health-Systems/Pages/default.aspx (accessed on June 17, 2022).

She added that additional research is needed to understand the interaction between application of the 4 Ms framework with race and ethnicity. A gradual approach that includes scaling up the mechanisms of the 4 Ms framework should decrease the likelihood of inadvertently building disparities into the system.

POLICY CHANGES TO MEET THE CHALLENGES OF CARING FOR PEOPLE WITH ADRD

Kate McEvoy, program officer Milbank Memorial Fund, began by describing several key considerations for improving the quality of care and supports for people with ADRD and their caregivers. She noted that efforts will require a focus on coordinating available resources at the local, state, and federal level for people with middle and low incomes. There are existing programs that have been created at the federal level to support improving quality of care for people with ADRD, such as the National Plan to Address Alzheimer's Disease.[5] There are also state-level programs, such as the Master Plan for Aging approach,[6] and the Older Americans Act (OAA) requires state plans for aging and state Alzheimer's disease plans (Colello and Napili, 2022).[7] There are also federal efforts to support access to care and services for people with ADRD, such as Aging and Disability Resource Centers and the No Wrong Door model.[8,9] Medicaid waiver supports and OAA National Family Caregiver (III-E) resources provide limited funding at the state level. There is an emerging evidence base in support of specific interventions, as well as the advancement of smart home and other technological approaches (Majumder et al., 2017).

McEvoy explained that despite these beneficial programs, challenges to progress remain. Federal and state planning, while effective, tends to be siloed. As an example, CMS and the Administration for Community Living (ACL) jointly manage Medicaid and OAA activities However, both could be more effective with better collaboration. Consumers are not adequately informed about resources such as Aging and Disability Resource Centers. This has led to

---

[5] See https://aspe.hhs.gov/collaborations-committees-advisory-groups/napa/napa-documents/napa-national-plans (accessed June 24, 2022).

[6] See https://www.thescanfoundation.org/publication-cat/master-plan-for-aging/ (accessed June 24, 2022).

[7] See https://alzimpact.org/media/serve/id/5d23af19258fb (accessed June 24, 2022).

[8] See https://acl.gov/programs/aging-and-disability-networks/aging-and-disability-resource-centers (accessed June 24, 2022).

[9] See https://acl.gov/programs/connecting-people-services/aging-and-disability-resource-centers-programno-wrong-door (accessed June 24, 2022).

such resources being underutilized until an individual experiences a crisis such as a fall or other hospitalization. She noted that care funding challenges, such as the lack of publicly funded and limited availability of commercial long-term care insurance, as well as variable access to Medicaid waivers for people living with ADRD, create additional barriers to improved care.

McEvoy offered three suggestions to address these challenges. First, CMS and ACL would benefit from improving coordination of their efforts through development of a joint framework for supporting people across the income and resource continuum. She emphasized that there is a need for improved consumer literacy about available benefits for ADRD care. Many people mistakenly believe that Medicare provides coverage for most long-term support services (LTSS). An effective approach for improving dissemination of information about resources such as Aging and Disability Resource Centers should include identifying messengers that community members consider trustworthy, including peers and physicians. She noted another opportunity for collaboration could be CMS endorsement of state Medicaid underwriting of Aging and Disability Resource Centers and services that support people with ADRD to live at home independently, such as home adaptation and tele-monitoring. Another strategy that could be implemented related to financing care for people with ADRD is to develop planning supports for people with ADRD that are spending down their financial resources to reach Medicaid eligibility. Her second suggestion was to create a publicly funded, payroll-based, long-term care insurance benefit. This benefit would defray the substantial out-of-pocket costs for ADRD care as well as serve as a vehicle for increasing consumer literacy about available benefits for ADRD care. Third, she noted that Medicaid could be enabled to have a greater effect on quality of care and supports for people with ADRD and their caregivers. She described several approaches that could better use Medicaid. These include a combined effort between Medicare and Medicaid to cover bundled payment models, such as Community Aging in Place-Advancing Better Living for Elders (CAPABLE[10]), and that include home care services, such as occupational therapy and home repair, and development of an LTSS Medicare/Medicaid waiver for people that are dually eligible that emphasizes coordinated care payments as well as measures directed at improving health equity and focuses on person-centered outcome measures. She also noted that legislative reforms, such as changing the statutory presumption that Medicaid is funding institutional care to a greater emphasis on funding home care and community-based services, could be beneficial. That approach could include making the Money Follows the Person demonstration project permanent.

---

[10] See https://nursing.jhu.edu/faculty_research/research/projects/capable/ (accessed July 29, 2022).

THE ROLE OF WORKFORCE ENGAGEMENT: LESSONS FROM NAPA

Helen Lamont, director, Division of Disability and Aging Policy, Department of Health and Human Services, Office of the Assistant Secretary for Planning and Evaluation (ASPE), began by discussing their work related to the National Alzheimer's Project Act (NAPA).[11] NAPA includes six goals:

1. Accelerating research to prevent and treat Alzheimer's disease
2. Optimizing care quality and efficiency
3. Expanding supports for people with Alzheimer's disease and their caregivers
4. Enhancing public awareness
5. Tracking progress
6. Promoting risk reduction.

Ten years after the inception of NAPA, Alzheimer's disease research funding has increased substantially. The Health Resources and Services Administration (HRSA) and ACL have expanded programs related to ADRD care, and policy makers have demonstrated increased engagement in efforts to improve ADRD care. She noted that ASPE's substantial collaboration efforts within and outside the federal government have been a major factor in NAPA's success. Another critical factor for NAPA's success has been the high level of commitment and expertise of the federal staff from all involved agencies.

Lamont next discussed the workforce involved in care of people with ADRD. She noted that this includes everyone involved with providing care and support for a person with ADRD, including health care providers and staff, community-based organizations and their staff, family caregivers, home care workers, and others. The ADRD care workforce faces a series of challenges. The demand for workers is growing as the population ages. People living with ADRD often have complicated chronic conditions and needs and may exhibit challenging behavioral and psychological symptoms. Providing care under those conditions can be emotionally and physically challenging as well as time consuming to coordinate. She noted that wages for direct care workers are not commensurate with the challenges associated with providing care for people with ADRD. This workforce has been heavily burdened during the COVID-19 pandemic, which exacerbated the existing challenges associated with providing care. The result was high rates of workforce turnover,

---

[11] See https://aspe.hhs.gov/collaborations-committees-advisory-groups/napa (accessed June 24, 2022).

labor shortages, increased costs, and poor quality of care, all of which make it difficult to implement new programs or initiatives related to quality of care.

Lamont emphasized the importance of the workforce tasked with providing direct care to people with ADRD. She noted that the 2022 National Academies of Sciences, Engineering, and Medicine consensus committee report addressing quality of care in nursing homes listed support for the workforce as its second goal, above financing reform (NASEM, 2022). Lamont opined that the most effective care is provided by an interprofessional team that brings together long-term care providers with other health care providers, which has implications for financing and how programs and policies are structured. She added that workforce education and engagement should be incorporated with payment policy changes to facilitate effective and sustainable strategies to improve quality of care and supports for people with ADRD.

DISCUSSION

Community Support for Sustainability

Faith Mitchell began by asking the group to discuss how behavioral change at the community level can increase sustainability of efforts for brain health. Lenz Lock explained that it is important for all communities, including the health care system, policy makers, and individuals, to understand that behavior change to promote brain health is possible and can have positive benefits. She added that each community needs to understand that they will benefit from improved brain health. For example, employers will reap the benefits of a healthier workforce that exercises regularly and receives adequate sleep. Health care providers that engage with their patients to encourage healthy behaviors that support brain health will also experience long-term benefits. Many people assume that deterioration and cognitive decline are inevitable aspects of aging, noted Mitchell. Lenz Lock noted that to combat this, AARP is working to engage people in an evidence-based brain health initiative.

The Role of Geriatricians in Promoting Adoption of the 4 Ms

Rebecca D. Alon, an audience member, asked the panel to discuss the role of geriatricians in supporting health care systems to adopt the 4 Ms model. Pelton began by explaining that the Age-Friendly Health Systems movement was developed to ensure that older adults, including those with ADRD,[12]

---

[12] See http://www.ihi.org/Engage/Initiatives/Age-Friendly-Health-Systems/Pages/default.aspx (accessed June 27, 2022).

receive evidence-based care, regardless of where in the health care system they are receiving care or whether a geriatrician is present. She added that one of the motivating factors for the development of the 4 Ms framework was to offer a guiding structure for care when there is not a geriatrician available, particularly given that not all health care facilities have geriatricians on staff. Hollmann noted that while it may not be feasible to have a geriatrician available to care for every older person, the American Geriatric Society has suggested that it would be appropriate for every Medicare Shared Savings Program to require somebody with geriatric expertise at a leadership level. He added that there is a precedent for this, as Medicare Part D plans are required to have a geriatrician and a geriatric pharmacologist as part of their organization.

Coordinating Federal Efforts

Gary Epstein-Lubow, Brown University, asked the group to discuss potential coordination among CDC, CMS, and ACL, particularly related to dissemination and implementation of evidence-based practices to improve quality of care for people living with ADRD. Lamont noted that implementation of the Building Our Largest Dementia (BOLD) Infrastructure for Alzheimer's Act began recently.[13] That includes coordination between the Aging Network and the public health networks.[14] She added that there is a BOLD Center of Excellence on Caregiving that is involved in efforts to disseminate programs operated by ACL. Lamont added that another opportunity would be greater collaborations between the Aging Network and the public health networks. She noted that there have been past efforts to combine Older Americans Act (OAA) services and Medicaid programs. She said that there is increasing interest in coordinating between agencies and suggested that efforts should avoid an excessive focus on cost-effectiveness that could create artificial barriers to improvement in quality of care. Lamont noted that it would be beneficial for OAA services to be viewed less as a means of reducing Medicaid expenditures and more as a strategy for supporting the segment of the population that is not eligible for Medicaid but requires support to continue to live in the community.

McEvoy noted that there may be unrealized opportunities for collaboration. Medicaid is very insular in its orientation to traditional services under state plans, but there are opportunities for specific intersections, such as Medicaid funding for Aging and Disability Resource Centers, which equip consumers to optimize their own resources under the ACL agenda. McEvoy noted

---

[13] See https://www.congress.gov/bill/115th-congress/senate-bill/2076 (accessed September 29, 2022).

[14] See https://eldercare.acl.gov/Public/About/Aging_Network/Index.aspx (accessed June 27, 2022).

some individual strands of funding have been less impactful than expected. She suggested that developing a strategy to combine those pieces could enable the states to do more, she said, noting that the COVID-19 pandemic created new opportunities for collaborations among health agencies.

Evaluation of Age Friendliness

Mitchell next asked Pelton how the effects of the age-friendly aspect of the 4 Ms framework could be distinguished from other factors that could affect patient outcomes. Pelton explained that they are evaluating the reach of the program by capturing the number of people who are reached by this care, as well as the effect of different aspects of the 4 Ms on outcomes, length of stay, and incidence of delirium. Pelton welcomed other interventions that have a positive effect on quality of care, such as the Age-Friendly Health System movement, geriatric emergency department (GED) accreditation, and geriatric surgery verification.[15] She explained that a critical component to support sustainable implementation is allowing space for individual health care systems to adapt the 4 Ms to their culture.

For example, in the Anne Arundel Medical Center, the "what matters" component of the 4 Ms demonstrated rapid uptake and was the catalyst for organizational change and adoption of the 4 Ms. The 4 Ms would not have been sustainably adopted at Anne Arundel had they not been given the flexibility to implement the program in a manner that fit their organization. She added that a combination of tools for quality improvement and autonomy for the care team have been important to facilitate broad and sustainable adoption of the 4 Ms framework. Lenz Lock noted that AARP has collaborated with USAging to develop a simple and inexpensive evaluation mechanism to determine whether the initiatives were effective for people with ADRD,[16] as well as the means to share successful practices. Lenz Lock encouraged communities to use these tools to share practices that lead to improved outcomes.

Engagement and Equity

Jennie Chin Hansen asked the group to discuss implementation of the 4 Ms in groups that have been historically made vulnerable and diverse populations. Pelton explained that Anne Arundel Medical Center, as well as

---

[15] See https://www.facs.org/quality-programs/accreditation-and-verification/geriatric-surgery-verification/ (accessed July 29, 2022).

[16] See https://www.usaging.org/dfa#:~:text=Through%20the%20collaborative%20efforts%20of,dementia%20and%20their%20care%20partners (accessed July 25, 2022).

another health care system in Michigan that implemented the 4 Ms framework, included substantial engagement with the communities they served and community-based services as part of their programming. She added that partnering with community-based organizations is a necessary part of the process, noting that UCLA and other systems have trained community health workers to use the 4 Ms framework. She also said that to ensure that sustainable practices are also equitable, outcomes should be measured by race and ethnicity. Mitchell noted that disparities in implementation of the 4 Ms related to race, ethnicity, and language barriers could be a concern. She added that community engagement is an important component of addressing those concerns.

Strategies to Support Remaining at Home

Emily Williams, an audience member, asked the group to discuss which services and supports they viewed as the most important to allow people with ADRD to remain in their homes and communities. Lenz Lock emphasized the importance of communicating with people about available supports and services. Lamont noted research that examined individual caregiver-related factors as predictors of a person being placed in a nursing home. She said that the strongest predictor was physical strains, such as falls or mobility limitations, night waking, and incontinence. She said another strong predictor was the behavioral and psychological symptoms of ADRD. Lamont said that addressing these challenges for caregivers requires a combination of physical supports and education. Pelton added that the most important approach is to identify the priorities of the person with ADRD and their family and organizing care around those priorities. McEvoy noted that changes to the traditional payment method for personal care supports under the home health model could be beneficial. She suggested one opportunity could be the development of an approach that accommodates reimbursement for services provided by a personal care assistant on an episodic basis. McEvoy added that another beneficial approach could be publicly funded respite benefits.

Education for Dementia Care and Brain Health

Audience member Gary Epstein-Lubow asked the group to discuss opportunities for collaboration on education efforts related to ADRD care and risk reduction. Lamont noted that HRSA's Geriatrics Workforce Enhancement Program has collaborated with ASPE and is disseminating information about best practices and evidence-based care. She added that some states provide geriatric or ADRD education to their workforces. She suggested that professional organizations should consider building education related to ADRD into their education requirements. She added that partnerships with non-governmental organizations are also essential to disseminating information.

McEvoy explained that during the COVID-19 pandemic, she noticed trusted sources of information for older adults and caregivers were not governments but peers and physicians, though the latter are not well equipped to act as advisors on complex issues of benefits and eligibility. Many communities chose to work through peer messengers and to tailor supports in ways that were culturally responsive and accessible to those that spoke languages other than English. She said that community health workers can act as trusted resources with lived experience for families experiencing ADRD. She recommended incorporating community health workers into value-based payment models. The federal government can be an incubator for these ideas.

Lamont noted that federal agencies could support innovation related to the incorporation of community health workers. She cited an example of a program funded by an ACL grant, the Wisconsin State Dementia Care Specialist program, through which community-based health providers deliver culturally responsive support for people with ADRD and their families. McEvoy noted that expert volunteers represent an untapped resource for supporting people with ADRD and their families. Lenz Lock suggested that a possible area for the National Institute on Aging (NIA) to research is how to develop a Medicare payment stream to support community-based organizations to provide services to people with ADRD, including training and partnership between the community-based organization (CBO) and health care providers.

Reducing the Burden on Primary Care Physicians

Hollmann asked the group to discuss strategies to develop tools that improve quality of care for people with ADRD while avoiding overburdening primary care providers. Lenz Lock noted that there is a need to develop a system that supports primary care providers referring people with ADRD to community-based organizations that could provide patient education. Pelton acknowledged the extra burden created by asking primary care physicians to engage in the 4 Ms. In the age-friendly health system movement, she said, she is working with regulators, policy makers, and accreditation bodies to identify opportunities to reduce workforce burden. Lamont added that technology, in the form of EHR alerts for providers, could also provide support to primary care providers.

7

Final Thoughts

At the conclusion of the workshop, Richard Frank asked speakers and moderators to reflect on key themes that had emerged over the course of the workshop. Terry Fulmer observed that the workshop represented a unique moment of a "confluence of ideas" about caring for people who are affected by Alzheimer's disease and related dementias (ADRD) from organizations such as government agencies, academic institutions, and national non-government organizations and foundations. She encouraged participants to offer their insights and research considerations, noting, "They [workshop sponsor NIA] are asking you, what is the scientific question in front of us that has to be answered in order to move this work [improving quality of care and supports for people living with ADRD and their caregivers] forward?"

CONSIDERING SUSTAINABILITY AND SCALING

Faith Mitchell began by stating that several presentations noted that while payment reform is necessary, it alone is not sufficient to bring about organizational behavioral change to improve quality of care and supports for people with ADRD and their caregivers. She highlighted the importance of sustainability, noting a need to determine how best to get individuals and systems to make long-term commitments to applying new models of care.

Terry Fulmer highlighted a need to engage experts in implementation science to more effectively translate research evidence into practice. She noted the Institute for Healthcare Improvement and the Education Development Center as examples of organizations with expertise in implementation science.[1] She said implementation science could be used to reliably translate research findings into practice in multiple settings related to ADRD care, including nursing homes and community-based care. She emphasized that systemic change must be based in science, including implementation science.

Julie Robison noted the role of supporting the health care workforce in scaling up effective models. She said several of the evidence-based models that have been effective, such as COPE and PACE, rely on being able to better pay and support the frontline workforce. She added better pay and support were also necessary to the success of the home- and community-based service programs that Kate McEvoy discussed.

SUPPORTING CAREGIVERS

Mitchell emphasized the need to support not just cost savings but quality of life for both person and caregiver so care can be provided effectively. She also noted that a recurring theme across presentations was that people living with ADRD are experiencing their disease within communities. This led her to suggest there is a need to better understand how to effectively use research to better support the role of the community in caring for people living with ADRD. Inouye called the billions of dollars spent by family caregivers in out-of-pocket expenses and lost work "just unconscionable in our country," and said she would like to see financial support for those caregivers. "We need more geriatricians and more home health care workers who are culturally sensitive and operating at the community level, but we are not realistically going to get those numbers, so we have to deputize our caregivers by providing them the training when they need it across the continuum of care," said Sarah Lenz Lock. She explained that training programs should prepare caregivers for what could be a 20-year disease course progressing from early-stage ADRD to end-stage ADRD.

Julie Robison drew on an example from cancer care to illustrate an opportunity to better support family caregivers. She noted that many cancer treatment programs include a patient navigator that is a paid member of the health care system. The patient navigator meets with patients diagnosed with cancer as well as their family caregivers and provides education about the diagnosis and treatment options as well as care coordination. She suggested that people diagnosed with ADRD and their caregivers would benefit from including paid patient navigators as part of ADRD care instead of as a separate service that requires out-of-pocket payment.

---

[1] See https://www.edc.org/.

QUALITY AND ACCOUNTABILITY: PREVENTING HARM

Inouye noted studies investigating potential models for ADRD care should also integrate quality measurement to support performance improvement and accountability. Frank, reflecting on the personal stories presented by workshop speakers, said, "We've got to stop doing bad stuff…that's at least a place to start." This is harm, said Fulmer, who encouraged NIA to fund efforts that engage implementation science to bring evidence-based care improvement into practice and reduce the excessive harm experienced by older people in the health care system. She cited the 2001 Institute of Medicine report, *Crossing the Quality Chasm: A New Health System for the 21st Century*, adding that the report could be applied to ADRD care (IOM, 2001).

Helen Lamont said it is shocking how few quality measures exist for the care of people with ADRD. She noted that diagnosis of ADRD when a person is in the early stages of their disease should be an expectation as well as a standard measure of quality. She added that early-stage diagnosis is currently neither an expectation nor a standard quality measure. She said that whether a home health aide appeared for a home visit is frequently considered a quality measurement for home- and community-based care, highlighting the need to address quality measures in home- and community-based services (HCBS) as well. She encouraged research to develop best practices for developing and implementing quality measures that set high standards for quality of care for people with ADRD throughout all phases of disease progression.

Lenz Lock highlighted the importance of changing expectations related to care for people with ADRD as a means of improving quality of care. She encouraged NIA to consider researching care approaches that focus on managing ADRD as a chronic disease with the potential for improved outcomes across the stages of disease progression. She emphasized an expectation that ADRD care could be and should be high quality, and development of evidence-based quality and outcome measures should lead to better care. She added that "stopping the bad stuff [poor quality care] starts with changing the expectation that it [poor quality care] will [happen]." She also encouraged moving away from the assumption that "an older person is frail and is going to fail," because that is not necessarily the case.

Robison noted another quality-related theme that appeared across workshop presentations is what matters to the person living with ADRD. She noted that quality care should be centered on what matters to the person living with ADRD. She said that what matters can change over the course of disease. She suggested more research is needed to determine how best to integrate the different components of what matters to that person into the different parts of their care throughout the progression of ADRD.

LONG-TERM CARE

Inouye encouraged making investigating effective payment models for long-term care, such as long-term care insurance, a higher priority. Lamont noted, "One fundamental truth about this population that came out is that they are one of the most vulnerable populations and they are sort of emblematic of everything you want in the entire health care system through the long-term care and end-of-life system." She said changing the health care system is a good starting point, but this should be integrated with changing long-term care systems, ensuring high-quality end-of-life care and improving support for caregivers. She added, "It is not just one organization's behavior change, it is changing this entire ecosystem and how we think really about health and well-being from our 40s on into the end of life." Lenz Lock agreed, adding, "The importance of thinking about this as a spectrum across a life span can't be overemphasized."

Robison called for more research focused on improving quality of care for people in the late and end stages of ADRD. She noted that Sherry mentioned during her presentation that the course of ADRD does not fit the trajectory of the current Medicare hospice benefit. Robison suggested research should be directed at improving the integration of palliative care and hospice care for people with ADRD as well as how best to incorporate what matters to patients into care for patients with late- and end-stage ADRD. She noted, there is also a need for a greater understanding of best approaches for preparing people diagnosed with ADRD and their families for the late and end stages of the disease.

CONSIDERING THE ROLE OF TECHNOLOGY

Robison noted Schneider's observations during his presentation about opportunities to use technology already in use in other industries to improve quality of care and supports for people living with ADRD and their caregivers. She encouraged research into possible cross-application of existing technology. She also suggested research to determine how to effectively incorporate technology and develop algorithms that can support primary care providers to create care plans for people with ADRD as well provide education for families. Lenz Lock noted that artificial intelligence (AI) was now being used to detect people who were likely to shoplift based on their gestures and other movements. She suggested another opportunity for additional research would be investigating the application of AI technology to predict and help older people who are about to fall. Frank suggested another opportunity for research could be related to incorporating smart home technology to better support people with ADRD.

EQUITY

Robison identified equity as an overarching theme of the workshop. She emphasized that ADRD does not affect all racial and ethnic groups the same. She said research funding priorities should reflect the need to keep equity central to the work of improving quality of care and support for people with ADRD and their caregivers. She suggested research efforts should emphasize who is most at risk of developing ADRD and who is most at risk of not receiving quality care or support for caregivers.

Mitchell also noted the overarching theme of equity. She recalled that Alzheimer's disease rates are twice as high in the Black community as in the White community, and that the Latinx community also has higher rates of the disease than the White community. She closed the discussion by asking, "All the way from mitigation to end of life, is it possible for us to address the needs of families and people living with Alzheimer's in ways that don't reinforce existing disparities in outcomes? So can we actually do things differently?"

Appendix A

References

AARP (American Association of Retired Persons). 2021. 2021 AARP survey on the perceptions related to a dementia diagnosis: Adults age 40-plus. *AARP Research.* https://www.aarp.org/content/dam/aarp/research/surveys_statistics/health/2021/dementia-diagnosis-perceptions.doi.10.26419-2Fres.00471.001.pdf (accessed July 28, 2022).

Alzheimer's Association. 2022. 2022 Alzheimer's disease facts and figures. *Alzheimer's & Dementia : The Journal of the Alzheimer's Association* 18(4):700-789.

American Medical Association. 2011. *Physician consortium for performance improvement (PCPI): Dementia performance measurement set.* Chicago, IL: AMA.

Anderson, T. S., E. R. Marcantonio, E. P. McCarthy, L. Ngo, M. A. Schonberg, and S. J. Herzig. 2022. Association of diagnosed dementia with post-discharge mortality and readmission among hospitalized Medicare beneficiaries. *Journal of General Internal Medicine.* https://doi.org/10.1007/s11606-022-07549-7.

Barber, S. L., K. van Gool, S. Wise, M. Woods, Z. Or, A. Penneau, R. Milstein, N. Ikegami, S. Kwon, P. Bakx, E. Schut, B. Wouterse, M. Flores, and L. Lorenzoni. 2021. *Pricing long-term care for older persons.* Geneva, Switzerland: World Health Organization and Organisation for Economic Co-operation and Development.

Barker, P. M., A. Reid, and M. W. Schall. 2016. A framework for scaling up health interventions: Lessons from large-scale improvement initiatives in Africa. *Implementation Science: IS* 11:12-12.

Belle, S. H., L. Burgio, R. Burns, D. Coon, S. J. Czaja, D. Gallagher-Thompson, L. N. Gitlin, J. Klinger, K. M. Koepke, C. C. Lee, J. Martindale-Adams, K. Nichols, R. Schulz, S. Stahl, A. Stevens, L. Winter, S. Zhang; MS for the Resources for Enhancing Alzheimer's Caregiver Health (REACH) II Investigators. 2006. Enhancing the quality of life of dementia caregivers from different ethnic or racial groups: A randomized, controlled trial. *Annals of Internal Medicine* 145(10):727-738.

Bindman, A. B., and D. F. Cox. 2018. Changes in health care costs and mortality associated with transitional care management services after a discharge among Medicare beneficiaries. *JAMA Internal Medicine* 178(9):1165-1171.

Boustani, M., C. A. Alder, C. A. Solid, and D. Reuben. 2019. An alternative payment model to support widespread use of collaborative dementia care models. *Health Affairs* 38(1):54-59.

Brookmeyer, R., N. Abdalla, C. H. Kawas, and M. M. Corrada. 2018. Forecasting the prevalence of preclinical and clinical Alzheimer's disease in the United States. *Alzheimers and Dementia Journal* 14(2):121-129.

Chang, C.-H., A. Mainor, S. Raymond, K. Peck, C. Colla, and J. Bynum. 2019. Inclusion of nursing homes and long-term residents in Medicare ACOs. *Medical Care* 57(12):990-995.

Chang, C. H., A. Mainor, C. Colla, and J. Bynum. 2021. Utilization by long-term nursing home residents under accountable care organizations. *Journal of American Medical Directors Association* 22(2):406-412.

Chi, W., E. Graf, L. Hughes, J. Hastie, G. Khatutsky, S. Shuman, E. A. Jessup, S. Karon, and H. Lamont. 2019. *Older adults with dementia and their caregivers: Key indicators from the National Health and Aging Trends Study.* Washington, DC: Office of the Assistant Secretary for Planning and Evaluation.

Clancy, C. 2019. Creating world-class care and service for our nation's finest: How Veterans Health Administration Diffusion of Excellence Initiative is innovating and transforming Veterans Affairs health care. *Permanente Journal* 23(4). https://doi.org/10.7812/TPP/18.301.

Clevenger, C. K., J. Cellar, M. Kovaleva, L. Medders, and K. Hepburn. 2018. Integrated memory care clinic: Design, implementation, and initial results. *Journal of the American Geriatrics Society* 66(12):2401-2407.

CMS (Centers for Medicare and Medicaid Services). 2018. *PACE quality monitoring integrated user guide.* https://www.npaonline.org/sites/default/files/PDFs/HPMS%20User%20Guide.pdf (accessed October 5, 2022).

CMS. 2021. *CMS funding 1,000 new residency slots for hospitals serving rural and underserved communities.* Washington, DC: U.S. Department of Health and Human Services.

CMS. 2022a. *CMS Fast Facts.* https://data.cms.gov/sites/default/files/2022-08/4f0176a6-d634-47c1-8447-b074f014079a/CMSFastFactsAug2022.pdf (accessed September 27, 2022).

CMS. 2022b. *CMS releases 2023 Medicare Advantage and Part D advance notice.* Washington, DC: U.S. Department of Health and Human Services..

CMS. 2022c. *Regulations and guidance.* https://www.cms.gov/Regulations-and-Guidance/Regulations-and-Guidance (accessed September 29, 2022).

Coe, N. B., and R. M. Werner. 2022. Informal caregivers provide considerable front-line support in residential care facilities and nursing homes. *Health Affairs* 41(1):105-111.

Colello, K. J., and A. Napili. 2022. *Older Americans Act: Overview and funding.* Washington, DC: Congressional Research Service.

Cornell, P. Y., W. Zhang, L. Smith, S. Fashaw, and K. S. Thomas. 2020. Developments in the market for assisted living: Residential care availability in 2017. *Journal of the American Medical Directors Association* 21(11):1718-1723.

De Vleminck, A., R. S. Morrison, D. E. Meier, and M. D. Aldridge. 2018. Hospice care for patients with dementia in the United States: A longitudinal cohort study. *Journal of the American Medical Directors Association* 19(7):633-638.

Feng, Z., J. Wang, A. Gadaska, M. Knowles, S. Haber, M. J. Ingber, and V. Grouverman. 2021. *Comparing outcomes for dual eligible beneficiaries in integrated care: Final report.* Washington, DC: RTI International for Office of Behavioral Health, Disability, and Aging Policy, Office of the Assistant Secretary for Planning and Evaluation, U.S. Department of Health and Human Services.

Fortinsky, R. H., L. N. Gitlin, L. T. Pizzi, C. V. Piersol, J. Grady, J. T. Robison, S. Molony, and D. Wakefield. 2020. Effectiveness of the Care of Persons with Dementia in their Environments intervention when embedded in a publicly funded home- and community-based service program. *Innovation in Aging* 4(6):igaa053.

French, D. D., M. A. LaMantia, L. R. Livin, D. Herceg, C. A. Alder, and M. A. Boustani. 2014. Healthy Aging Brain Center improved care coordination and produced net savings. *Health Affairs* 33(4):613-618.

Fulmer, T., L. Pelton, J. Zhang, and W. Huang, eds. 2022. *Age-friendly health systems: A guide to using the 4 Ms while caring for older adults.* Boston, MA: Institute for Healthcare Improvement.

Garfield, R., M. Musumeci, E. L. Reavers, and A. Damico. 2015. *Medicaid's role for people with dementia.* San Francisco, CA: Henry J. Kaiser Family Foundation.

Gaugler, J. E., M. Reese, and M. S. Mittelman. 2018. Process evaluation of the NYU caregiver intervention-adult child. *Gerontologist* 58(2):e107-e117.

Gitlin, L. N., L. Winter, M. P. Dennis, N. Hodgson, and W. W. Hauck. 2010. A biobehavioral home-based intervention and the well-being of patients with dementia and their caregivers: The COPE randomized trial. *JAMA* 304(9):983-991.

GCBH (Global Council on Brain Health). 2022. *CHOOSE Brain-Healthy Habits.* https://www.aarp.org/content/dam/aarp/health/brain_health/2022-03/gcbh-behavior-change-infographic-english.doi.10.26419-2Fpia.00106.002.pdf (accessed July 28, 2022). https://doi.org/ss26419/pia.00106.002

Grabowski, D. C. 2007. Medicare and Medicaid: Conflicting incentives for long-term care. *Milbank Quarterly* 85(4):579-610.

Gupta, Reshma, L. Roh, C. Lee, D. Reuben, A. Naeim, J. Wilson, and S. A. Skootsky. 2019. The population health value framework: Creating value by reducing costs of care for patient subpopulations with chronic conditions. *Academic Medicine* 94(9):1337-1342. https://doi.org/10.1097/ACM.0000000000002739.

Haggerty, K. L., G. Epstein-Lubow, L. H. Spragens, R. J. Stoeckle, L. C. Evertson, L. A. Jennings, and D. B. Reuben. 2020. Recommendations to improve payment policies for comprehensive dementia care. *Journal of the American Geriatrics Society* 68(11):2478-2485.

Hiyoshi-Taniguchi, K., C. B. Becker, and A. Kinoshita. 2018. What behavioral and psychological symptoms of dementia affect caregiver burnout? *Clinical Gerontology* 41(3):249-254.

Hurd, M. D., P. Martorell, A. Delavande, K. J. Mullen, and K. M. Langa. 2013. Monetary costs of dementia in the United States. *New England Journal of Medicine* 368(14):1326-1334.

Hwang, U., C. Carpenter, S. Dresden, J. Dussetschleger, A. Gifford, L. Hoang, J. Leggett, A. Nowroozpoor, Z. Taylor, M. Shah; Gear*, and G. Networks. 2022. The geriatric emergency care applied research (GEAR) network approach: A protocol to advance stakeholder consensus and research priorities in geriatrics and dementia care in the emergency department. *BMJ Open* 12(4):e060974.

IOM (Institute of Medicine). 1986. *Improving the quality of care in nursing homes.* Washington, DC: National Academy Press.

IOM Committee on Quality of Health Care in America. 2001. *Crossing the quality chasm: A new health system for the 21st century.* Washington, DC: National Academy Press.

Jaeger-Fine, T. M. 2020. U.S. Administrative Law. In *American Legal Systems,* 3rd ed. Durham, NC: Carolina Academic Press. Pp. 55-66.

Jennings, L. A., Z. Tan, N. S. Wenger, E. A. Cook, W. Han, H. E. McCreath, K. S. Serrano, C. P. Roth, and D. B. Reuben. 2016. Quality of care provided by a comprehensive dementia care comanagement program. *Journal of the American Geriatrics Society* 64(8):1724-1730.

JAF (John A. Hartford Foundation). 2018. *Discovering the 4 Ms: A Framework for Creating Age-Friendly Health Systems.* https://www.johnahartford.org/blog/view/discovering-the-4ms-a-framework-for-creating-age-friendly-health-systems/ (accessed September 29, 2022).

Johnson, R. W., and S. Lindner. 2016. *Older adults' living expenses and the adequacy of income allowances for Medicaid home and community-based services.* Washington, DC: U.S. Department of Health and Human Services, Office of the Assistant Secretary for Planning and Evaluation.

Jutkowitz, E., R. L. Kane, J. E. Gaugler, R. F. MacLehose, B. Dowd, and K. M. Kuntz. 2017. Societal and family lifetime cost of dementia: Implications for policy. *Journal of the American Geriatrics Society* 65(10):2169-2175.

Kellett, K., K. Ligus, and J. Robison. 2021. "So glad to be home": Money Follows the Person participants' experiences after transitioning out of an institution. *Journal of Disability Policy Studies* 33(2):122-132. https://doi.org/10.1177/10442073211043519.

Kellett, K., J. Robison, H. McAbee-Sevick, L. N. Gitlin, C. Verrier Piersol, and R. H. Fortinsky. 2022. Implementing the Care of Persons with Dementia in their Environments (COPE) intervention in community-based programs: Acceptability and perceived benefit from care managers' and interventionists' perspectives. *Gerontologist* gnac068. https://doi.org/10.1093/geront/gnac068.

Kennedy, M., A. Lesser, J. Israni, S. W. Liu, I. Santangelo, N. Tidwell, L. T. Southerland, C. R. Carpenter, K. Biese, S. Ahmad, and U. Hwang. 2022. Reach and adoption of a geriatric emergency department accreditation program in the United States. *Annals of Emergency Medicine* 79(4):367-373.

Knox, S., B. Downer, A. Haas, A. Middleton, and K. J. Ottenbacher. 2020a. Dementia severity associated with increased risk of potentially preventable readmissions during home health care. *Journal of the American Medical Directors Association* 21(4):519-524.e513.

Knox, S., B. Downer, A. Haas, A. Middleton, and K. J. Ottenbacher. 2020b. Function and caregiver support associated with readmissions during home health for individuals with dementia. *Archives of Physical Medicine and Rehabilitation* 101(6):1009-1016.

Korthauer, L. E., C. Denby, D. Molina, J. Wanjiku, L. A. Daiello, J. D. Drake, J. D. Grill, and B. R. Ott. 2021. Pilot study of an Alzheimer's disease risk assessment program in a primary care setting. *Alzheimer's & Dementia: Diagnosis, Assessment & Disease Monitoring* 13(1):e12157.

Lang, L., A. Clifford, L. Wei, D. Zhang, D. Leung, G. Augustine, I. M. Danat, W. Zhou, J. R. Copeland, K. J. Anstey, and R. Chen. 2017. Prevalence and determinants of undetected dementia in the community: A systematic literature review and a meta-analysis. *BMJ Open* 7(2):e011146.

Langley, G. L., R. Moen, K. M. Nolan, T. W. Nolan, C. L. Norman, and L. P. Provost. 2009. *The Improvement Guide: A practical approach to enhancing organizational performance.* 2nd ed. San Francisco, CA: Jossey-Bass Publishers.

Larson, E. B., M. F. Shadlen, L. Wang, W. C. McCormick, J. D. Bowen, L. Teri, and W. A. Kukull. 2004. Survival after initial diagnosis of Alzheimer's disease. *Annals of Internal Medicine* 140(7):501-509.

Lees Haggerty, K., G. Epstein-Lubow, L. H. Spragens, R. J. Stoeckle, L. C. Evertson, L. A. Jennings, and D. B. Reuben. 2020. Recommendations to improve payment policies for comprehensive dementia care. *Journal of the American Geriatrics Society* 68(11):2478-2485.

Li, J., C. Andy, and S. Mitchell. 2021. Use of Medicare's new reimbursement codes for cognitive assessment and care planning, 2017-2018. *JAMA Network Open* 4(9):e2125725.

Livingston, G., J. Huntley, A. Sommerlad, D. Ames, C. Ballard, S. Banerjee, C. Brayne, A. Burns, J. Cohen-Mansfield, C. Cooper, S. G. Costafreda, A. Dias, N. Fox, L. N. Gitlin, R. Howard, H. C. Kales, M. Kivimäki, E. B. Larson, A. Ogunniyi, V. Orgeta, K. Ritchie, K. Rockwood, E. L. Sampson, Q. Samus, L. S. Schneider, G. Selbæk, L. Teri, and N. Mukadam. 2020. Dementia prevention, intervention, and care: 2020 report of the Lancet Commission. *Lancet* 396(10248):413-446.

Majumder, S., E. Aghayi, M. Noferesti, H. Memarzadeh-Tehran, T. Mondal, Z. Pang, and M. J. Deen. 2017. Smart homes for elderly healthcare: Recent advances and research challenges. *Sensors (Basel, Switzerland)* 17(11):2496.

Marrero, J., R. H. Fortinsky, G. A. Kuchel, and J. Robison. 2019. Risk factors for falls among older adults following transition from nursing home to the community. *Medical Care Research and Review* 76(1):73-88.

Masters, M. C., J. C. Morris, and C. M. Roe. 2015. "Noncognitive" symptoms of early Alzheimer's disease: A longitudinal analysis. *Neurology* 84(6):617-622.

Mate, K., T. Fulmer, L. Pelton, A. Berman, A. Bonner, W. Huang, and J. Zhang. 2021. Evidence for the 4 Ms: Interactions and outcomes across the care continuum. *Journal of Aging and Health* 33(7-8):469-481.

Mathematica. 2017. Research and evaluation of the Money Follows the Person (MFP) demonstration grants. https://www.mathematica.org/projects/research-and-evaluation-of-the-money-follows-the-person-mfp-demonstration-grants (accessed June 10, 2022).

Maughan, B. C., D. C. Kahvecioglu, G. Marrufo, G. M. Gerding, S. Dennen, J. K. Marshall, D. M. Cooper, C. M. Kummet, and L. A. Dummit. 2019. Medicare's Bundled Payments for Care Improvement initiative maintained quality of care for vulnerable patients. *Health Affairs* 38(4):561-568.

McDade, E., M. M. Bednar, H. R. Brashear, D. S. Miller, P. Maruff, C. Randolph, Z. Ismail, M. C. Carrillo, C. J. Weber, L. J. Bain, and A. M. Hake. 2020. The pathway to secondary prevention of Alzheimer's disease. *Alzheimers and Dementia Journal* 6(1):e12069. https://doi.org/10.1002/trc2.12069.

McNab, J., and J. A. Gillespie. 2015. Bridging the chronic care gap: HealthOne Mt Druitt, Australia. *International Journal of Integrated Care* 15:e015.

NASEM (National Academies of Sciences, Engineering, and Medicine). 2022. *The national imperative to improve nursing home quality: Honoring our commitment to residents, families, and staff.* Washington, DC: The National Academies Press.

Pangman, V. C., J. Sloan, and L. Guse. 2000. An examination of psychometric properties of the Mini-Mental State Examination and the Standardized Mini-Mental State Examination: Implications for clinical practice. *Applied Nursing Research* 13(4):209-213.

Perlo, J., B. Balik, S. Swensen, A. Kabcenell, and D. Feeley. 2017. *IHI framework for improving joy in work.* IHI white paper. Cambridge, MA: Institute for Healthcare Improvement.

Pizzi, L. T., E. Jutkowitz, K. M. Prioli, E. Y. Lu, Z. Babcock, H. McAbee-Sevick, D. B. Wakefield, J. Robison, S. Molony, C. V. Piersol, L. N. Gitlin, and R. H. Fortinsky. 2022. Cost-benefit analysis of the COPE program for persons living with dementia: Toward a payment model. *Innovation in Aging* 6(1):igab042.

Rapp, S. R., and D. Chao. 2000. Appraisals of strain and of gain: Effects on psychological well-being of caregivers of dementia patients. *Aging & Mental Health* 4(2):142-147.

Reuben, D. B., Z. S. Tan, T. Romero, N. S. Wenger, E. Keeler, and L. A. Jennings. 2019. Patient and caregiver benefit from a comprehensive dementia care program: 1-year results from the UCLA Alzheimer's and dementia care program. *Journal of the American Geriatrics Society* 67(11):2267-2273.

Robison, J., M. Porter, N. Shugrue, A. Kleppinger, and D. Lambert. 2015. Connecticut's "money follows the person" yields positive results for transitioning people out of institutions. *Health Affairs* 34(10):1628-1636.

Robison, J., N. Shugrue, M. Porter, and K. Baker. 2020. Challenges to community transitions through Money Follows the Person. *Health Services Research* 55(3):357-366.

Robison, J. T., N. A. Shugrue, R. H. Fortinsky, C. D. Fabius, K. Baker, M. Porter, and J. J. Grady. 2021. A new stage of the caregiving career: Informal caregiving after long-term institutionalization. *Gerontologist* 61(8):1211-1220.

Ryan, J., and B. C. Edwards. 2015. Health policy brief: Rebalancing Medicaid long-term services and supports. *Health Affairs* September 17. https://doi.org/10.1377/hpb20150917.439553.

Ryman, D. C., N. Acosta-Baena, P. S. Aisen, T. Bird, A. Danek, N. C. Fox, A. Goate, P. Frommelt, B. Ghetti, J. B. Langbaum, F. Lopera, R. Martins, C. L. Masters, R. P. Mayeux, E. McDade, S. Moreno, E. M. Reiman, J. M. Ringman, S. Salloway, P. R. Schofield, R. Sperling, P. N. Tariot, C. Xiong, J. C. Morris, and R. J. Bateman. 2014. Symptom onset in autosomal dominant alzheimer disease: A systematic review and meta-analysis. *Neurology* 83(3):253-260.

Savva, G. M., and A. Arthur. 2015. Who has undiagnosed dementia? A cross-sectional analysis of participants of the Aging, Demographics and Memory study. *Age and Ageing* 44(4):642-647.

Schurrer, J., A. O'Malley, C. Wilson, N. McCall, and N. Jain. 2017. *Evaluation of the diffusion and impact of the Chronic Care Management (CCM) services: Final report.* Princeton, NJ: Mathematica Policy Research.

Seshamani, M., and D. B. Jacobs. 2022. Leveraging Medicare to advance health equity. *JAMA* 327(18):1757-1758.

Seshamani, M., E. Fowler, and C. Brooks-LaSure. 2022. Building on the CMS strategic vision: Working together for a stronger Medicare. *Health Affairs Forefront.* https://www.healthaffairs.org/do/10.1377/forefront.20220110.198444 (accessed July 29, 2022).

Sharkey, T. 2017. Mental health strategy and impact evaluation in QATAR. *BJPsych International* 14(1):18-21.

Wagner, E. H., K. Coleman, R. J. Reid, K. Phillips, M. K. Abrams, and J. R. Sugarman. 2012. The changes involved in patient-centered medical home transformation. *Primary Care* 39(2):241–259. https://doi.org/10.1016/j.pop.2012.03.002.

Wagner, E. H., R. Gupta, and K. Coleman. 2014. Practice transformation in the Safety Net Medical Home initiative: A qualitative look. *Medical Care* 52(11 Suppl 4):S18-S22. https://doi.org/10.1097/MLR.0000000000000196.

Wang, J., T. V. Caprio, A. Simning, J. Shang, Y. Conwell, F. Yu, and Y. Li. 2020. Association between home health services and facility admission in older adults with and without Alzheimer's disease. *Journal of the American Medical Directors Association* 21(5):627-633.e629.

Wang, S., D. Yan, H. Temkin-Greener, and S. Cai. 2021. Nursing home admissions for persons with dementia: Role of home- and community-based services. *Health Services Research* 56(6):1168-1178.

Wenger, N. S., C. P. Roth, P. Shekelle, and ACOVE Investigators. 2007. Introduction to the Assessing Care of Vulnerable Elders-3 quality indicator measurement set. *Journal of the American Geriatrics Society* 55:S247-S252.

Werner, R. M., and E. Bressman. 2021. Trends in post-acute care utilization during the COVID-19 pandemic. *Journal of the American Medical Directors Association* 22(12):2496-2499.

WHO (World Health Organization). 2015. *World report on ageing and health.* Geneva, Switzerland: World Health Organization.

WHO. 2017. *Global action plan on the public health response to dementia 2017–2025.* Geneva, Switzerland: World Health Organization.

WHO. 2021. *Framework for countries to achieve an integrated continuum of long-term care.* Geneva, Switzerland: World Health Organization.

WHO. 2022. *Integrated Care for Older People (ICOPE) implementation pilot programme: Findings from the 'ready' phase.* Geneva, Switzerland: World Health Organization.

Appendix B

Statement of Task

The National Academies of Sciences, Engineering, and Medicine project staff from the Board on Health Care Services in collaboration with the Board on Behavioral, Cognitive, and Sensory Sciences will undertake all activities necessary for a 2-day public workshop to explore mechanisms that might improve care to meet the needs of people living with Alzheimer's disease and related dementias (ADRD), connected to sustainable payment models that can be adopted by organizations. While many health systems, public health, and social service systems are redesigning their programs and processes to address the current siloed nature of care and service delivery, there remains a gap in understanding how to reliably implement organizational behavior change initiatives to better serve people living with ADRD. Possible health outcomes and care processes that may be explored as highly responsive to hospital organizational behavioral changes include

- health care-associated infections;
- in-facility safety (mobility promotion, fall prevention, physical restraints);
- mentation management services (evaluating and addressing psychological and psychiatric symptoms);
- care transitions (including medication reconciliation); and
- person-centered care (assessments of what matters to people living with ADRD, including person-centered care goals and advance care planning).

A planning committee of the National Academies of Sciences, Engineering, and Medicine will define the specific topics to be addressed, develop the agenda, and select and invite speakers and other participants. After the workshop, a proceedings of the workshop will be prepared by a rapporteur, reviewed according to National Academies' report review procedures, and publicly released on the National Academies Press website. Background materials distributed for the workshop, presentation slides, and the like will be made available on the National Academies' website.

Appendix C

Workshop Agenda

Day 1
May 23, 2022
9:00 am ET–4:10 pm ET

9:00 am **Welcome and Workshop Overview**
Richard Frank, Planning Committee Chair, USC–Brookings Schaeffer Initiative on Health Policy

Sponsor Remarks from NIA
Melinda Kelley, National Institute on Aging at the National Institutes of Health

9:20 am **Keynotes**
Keynote Speakers:
David Reuben, University of California, Los Angeles
Meena Seshamani, Center for Medicare

10:10 am **Break**

10:25 am **Session 1 Defining Quality**
Moderator:
Terry Fulmer, the John A. Hartford Foundation

Speakers:
- Betty Ferrell, City of Hope
- Eric Schneider, National Committee for Quality Assurance
- Lisa Gwyther, Duke University

Followed by moderated discussion

11:55 am   **Lunch**

12:55 pm   **Session 2 Transforming the Role of Payment System Incentives to Improve Quality**
Moderator:
Richard Frank, USC–Brookings Schaeffer Initiative on Health Policy
Speakers:
- Tisamarie Sherry, Office of the Assistant Secretary for Planning and Evaluation, U.S. Department of Health and Human Services
- Bruce Vladeck, Greater New York Hospital Association, LiveOnNY
- Emily Largent, Penn IMPACT Ethics Core, University of Pennsylvania
- Amol Navathe, Penn Center for Health Incentives and Behavioral Economics, University of Pennsylvania

Followed by moderated discussion

2:25 pm   **Break**

2:40 pm   **Session 3 Evidence on Impact of Existing Models and Research and Innovation to Address Gaps in Data and Evidence**
Moderator:
Sharon Inouye, Harvard Medical School
Speakers:
- Julie Robison, University of Connecticut
- Peter Hollmann, Brown University, Lifespan Health Alliance Medicare ACO
- Hyobum Jang, World Health Organization
- Jennie Chin Hansen, SCAN Healthcare

Followed by moderated discussion

APPENDIX C

4:10 pm   **Adjourn for the day**

Day 2
May 24, 2022
9:30 am ET–12:00 pm ET

9:30 am   **Session 4 Creating Change**
Moderator:
Faith Mitchell, the Urban Institute
Speakers:
- Leslie Pelton, Institute for Healthcare Improvement
- Sarah Lock, AARP, Global Council on Brain Health
- Kate McEvoy, Milbank Memorial Fund
- Helen Lamont, Office of the Assistant Secretary for Planning and Evaluation, U.S. Department of Health and Human Services

Followed by moderated discussion

11:00 am   **Break**

11:15 am   **Planning Committee Discussion**

11:55 am   **Closing Remarks**

Appendix D

Biographical Sketches of the Speakers and Committee Members

BIOGRAPHICAL SKETCHES OF THE SPEAKERS

Betty Ferrell, R.N., Ph.D., M.A., CHPN, FAAN, FPCN, has been in nursing for 44 years and has focused her clinical expertise and research in pain management, quality of life, and palliative care. Dr. Ferrell is the director of nursing research and education and a professor at the City of Hope Medical Center in Duarte, California. She is a fellow of the American Academy of Nursing, and she has more than 480 publications in peer-reviewed journals and texts. She is principal investigator of the End-of-Life Nursing Education Consortium (ELNEC) project. She directs several other funded projects related to palliative care in cancer centers and quality-of-life issues. Dr. Ferrell was cochairperson of the National Consensus Project for Quality Palliative Care. Dr. Ferrell completed a master's degree in theology, ethics, and culture from Claremont Graduate University in 2007. She has authored 11 books, including the Oxford *Textbook of Palliative Nursing* (5th edition, 2019) published by Oxford University Press. She is coauthor of the text, *The Nature of Suffering and the Goals of Nursing* (Oxford University Press, 2008) and *Making Health Care Whole: Integrating Spirituality into Patient Care* (Templeton Press, 2010). In 2013 Dr. Ferrell was named one of the 30 visionaries in the field by the American Academy of Hospice and Palliative Medicine. In 2019 she was elected a member of the National Academy of Medicine. In 2021 Dr. Ferrell received the Oncology Nursing Society Lifetime Achievement Award, and she was inducted as a Living Legend by the American Academy of Nursing.

Lisa Gwyther, M.S.W., LCSW is a clinical social worker with 42 years of experience working with older adults and dementia-specific services. She is an associate professor emerita at the Duke School of Medicine's Department of Psychiatry and Behavioral Sciences, and a senior fellow at Duke University's Center for Aging. Ms. Gwyther is the founding director (1980) of the Duke Dementia Family Support Program, a community-based program offering education, consultation, support, and engagement opportunities for individuals living with dementia, their families, and the professionals serving them. Program services are provided at no cost and are not limited to Duke patients. Ms. Gwyther was principal investigator for education, minority engagement, and outreach for an NIA Alzheimer's Disease Research Center at Duke from 1985 to 2011. Her 160 peer-reviewed research articles, books, award-winning documentary films, and book chapters focus on developing and testing effective educational and support strategies targeting individuals living with dementia and their families to improve the quality of care and decision-making for individuals while reducing the negative health, emotional, and financial consequences for families providing that care. Ms. Gwyther served on two recent American Bar Association (ABA) panels representing interests of families of persons living with dementia, and she currently serves on the ABA Commission on Law and Aging. She was a consensus panelist on the National Academies of Sciences, Engineering, and Medicine 2016 report, *Families Caring for an Aging America*, and she co-chaired the North Carolina 2016 Dementia-Capable NC State Plan. Ms. Gwyther was the first John Heinz Congressional Fellow in Health and Aging, and she served for nine years on the first U.S. federal Alzheimer's Advisory Panel. Ms. Gwyther was named the 2019 NC Pioneer in Aging by the NC Coalition on Aging representing all state aging services, policy, and advocacy organizations. She is a former president of the Gerontological Society of America.

Jennie Chin Hansen, M.S., is the immediate past CEO of the American Geriatrics Society, the largest professional membership organization of geroclinicians committed to the care of older adults living with care complexity. Prior to this position she completed her role as president of the 38 million member AARP during the negotiations and development of the Affordable Care Act. She currently contributes in content areas of dementia, workforce, chronic complex care, and health equity. Her primary career includes nearly 25 years in San Francisco providing integrated, globally financed, and comprehensive medical and community-based service, including home care sites for nursing home–eligible older persons. Its groundbreaking fully capitated, integrated, and coordinated service delivery system became the prototype for the 1997 federal law that established the Program of All Inclusive Care for the Elderly (PACE) into the Medicare and Medicaid programs. PACE now operates extensively in California and in 30 other states. She has served as a federal commissioner on MedPAC (Medicare policy and payment) and serves or has served on several boards related to health care and philanthropy (including 12 years on the SCAN Foundation). In 2021 she completed her formal role as one of the stakeholders who crafted the first ever California MasterPlan for Aging.

Peter Hollmann, M.D., is chief medical officer for Brown Medicine, the practice group of the Brown University, Warren Alpert School of Medicine Department of Medicine. Until 2015, he was associate chief medical officer for Blue Cross & Blue Shield of Rhode Island. He has a part-time geriatric primary care practice in Rhode Island. He has more than 30 years of experience in medical management, including as a medical director of a health maintenance organization (HMO) with a Medicare product, a Medicaid plan, and a commercial preferred provider organization (PPO). He has been a long-term care hospital, nursing home, home care, and Medicare shared savings program ACO medical director. He chairs the American Geriatrics Society (AGS) committee that works on the Medicare Physician Fee Schedule, is a member of the AGS Beers criteria panel, and is the AGS board chair. He has been active in creating geriatric measures for Medicare and the National Center for Quality Assurance. He is past chair of the CPT Editorial Panel and currently vice chair of the resource-based relative value scale (RBRVS) Update Committee. He is chair of the Health Resources and Services Administration (HRSA) Council on Graduate Medical Education (COGME). His major duties presently involve practice transformation, development of systems of care, and population management. Much of his career has been devoted to quality improvement at the local and national level.

Hyobum Jang, M.D., M.P.H., is the technical officer responsible for long-term care in the Ageing and Health Unit at the World Health Organization. Dr. Jang joined WHO in 2015 and has worked at global, regional, and country levels, in the Philippines, Samoa, and Fiji, and now WHO headquarters in Geneva, Switzerland. His professional experience covers a wide range of health program areas, including community-based primary health care, noncommunicable diseases, climate change and health, sexual and reproductive health and rights, and most recently healthy aging and long-term care. Dr. Jang received his medical degree from Seoul University College of Medicine and his master's degree in public health from Harvard School of Public Health.

Helen Lamont Ph.D. is the director of the Division of Disability and Aging Policy, where she manages a team of professional staff that conduct policy analysis, research, and evaluation related to disability, aging, and long-term care issues and programs. Helen also leads the implementation of the National

Alzheimer's Project Act, coordinating both the Advisory Council on Alzheimer's Research, Care, and Services as well as an interagency group that writes the annual National Plan to Address Alzheimer's Disease. Helen also leads a portfolio of research in dementia, including a project to examine use of inpatient psychiatric facilities by people with dementia. She works on family and informal caregiving, as well as elder justice and adult maltreatment. Helen has worked across the department on disability data issues and has a current project to explore the feasibility of using an internet panel study to collect data on disability. She joined Office of the Assistant Secretary for Planning and Evaluation in 2007 and has a Ph.D. in aging studies from the University of South Florida and a B.S. in human development from Duke University.

Emily Largent, J.D., Ph.D., R.N., is the Emanuel and Robert Hart Assistant Professor of Medical Ethics and Health Policy; she holds a secondary appointment at Penn Law. Dr. Largent's work explores ethical and regulatory aspects of human subjects research and the translation of research findings into care with a particular focus on Alzheimer's disease and the patient–caregiver dyad. Her research is supported by the National Institute on Aging and the Greenwall Foundation.

Sarah Lenz Lock, J.D., is senior vice president for policy and brain health in AARP's Policy, Research, and International Affairs Department. Ms. Lock leads AARP's policy initiatives on brain health and care for people living with dementia, including serving as the executive director of the Global Council on Brain Health, an independent collaborative of scientists, doctors, and policy experts. Ms. Lock also coordinates AARP's role in the Leadership Council of Aging Organizations. Previously at AARP, Ms. Lock directed the Office of Policy Development and Integration, where she led the office responsible for the development of AARP's public policies. Her first role at AARP was as a senior attorney/manager at AARP Foundation Litigation conducting health care impact litigation on behalf of older persons. She has authored numerous amicus briefs in appellate courts all over the country on health care issues affecting older Americans. Ms. Lock is a frequent writer and public speaker on issues related to healthy aging. She has been quoted or appeared in numerous media outlets, including the *New York Times*, *NPR*, the *Washington Post*, the *Wall Street Journal*, *CBS News*, the *Baltimore Sun,* and the *Chicago Tribune.*

Kate McEvoy, J.D., is a program officer for the Milbank Memorial Fund. In this capacity, she leads the Fund's state leadership programs and network and guides the Fund's healthy aging work. Ms. McEvoy was previously director of health services in the Connecticut Department of Social Services, where she oversaw care delivery and payment reform work in Medicaid, CHIP, and long-term services and supports. She is a former president and vice president of the National Association of Medicaid Directors Board of Directors and served on the steering committee of the Reforming States Group, the predecessor to the Milbank State Leadership Network. She also contributed to state health reform initiatives as assistant comptroller for the State of Connecticut. An elder law attorney by training, Ms. McEvoy spent her early career working for a regional Agency on Aging and as a legislative liaison for the Connecticut Association of Area Agencies on Aging. She is a past chair of the Elder Law Section of the Connecticut Bar Association, is the author of a treatise on elder law, and led several major coalition-based projects around advance directives. She has a J.D. from the University of Connecticut School of Law and a B.A. in English and economics from Oberlin College.

Amol Navathe, M.D., Ph.D., is codirector of the Healthcare Transformation Institute and director of the Payment Insights Team at the University of Pennsylvania, where he is also an associate director of the Center for Health Incentives and Behavioral Economics. He is also physician and core investigator at the Philadelphia Veterans Affairs Medical Center. He is a commissioner of the Medicare Payment Advisory Commission, a nonpartisan agency that advises the U.S. Congress on Medicare policy, and he serves as an advisor to the governments of Singapore and Canada on health care financing and delivery models. Dr. Navathe is also a cofounder of Embedded Healthcare, a health care technology company that brings behavioral economics solutions to improving health care affordability and quality.

Dr. Navathe is a leading scholar on payment model design and evaluation, particularly bundled payments. His scholarship is unique because of its bi-directional translation between scientific discovery and real-world practice, including focus on (1) the impact of value-based care and payment models on health care value; (2) financial and nonfinancial incentive design, including applications of behavioral economics, to drive clinician practice change; and (3) a mix of pragmatic clinical trials and observational data analyses. He has published over 100 peer-reviewed articles in *Science*, the *New England Journal of Medicine*, the *Journal of the American Medical Association (JAMA)*, *Health Affairs*, and other leading journals, as well as the *New York Times* and other news outlets. Dr. Navathe completed medical school at the University of Pennsylvania School of Medicine and internal medicine residency at the Brigham and Women's Hospital at Harvard Medical School. He obtained his Ph.D. in Health Care Management and Economics from the Wharton School at the University of Pennsylvania.

Leslie Pelton, M.P.A., is an outcome-oriented leader who catalyzes innovation in health systems and transforms passion into impactful action. Throughout her 24-year career, Leslie has brought these talents to the improvement of health and health care of adults of all ages in community, health care practice, hospital, and nursing home–based care. Leslie listens deeply to the challenges that executives and frontline teams face. She collaboratively designs responses and leads the application of improvement science to build on will and drive improved outcomes.

Leslie is a nationally recognized leader in the Age-Friendly Health Systems movement improving the health and health care of older adults across the United States. With funders, national partners, leading health systems, and the Institute for Healthcare Improvement team, she designed the campaign that has resulted in improved care of older adults in 1,000 places of care across the United States. Throughout her career, Leslie has consulted with major academic medical centers, including building new models of integrating research, clinical care, and policy resulting in improved outcomes. She built and led her own consulting firm and served as faculty for the Institute for Healthcare Improvement. Leslie also built a practice at Deloitte Consulting addressing the human factors associated with strategy and operational innovations.

David B. Reuben, M.D., is the director, Multicampus Program in Geriatrics Medicine and Gerontology, and chief, Division of Geriatrics at the University of California, Los Angeles (UCLA) Center for Health Sciences. He is the Archstone Foundation chair and professor at the David Geffen School of Medicine at UCLA and director of the UCLA Alzheimer's and Dementia Care Program. Dr. Reuben is a past president of the American Geriatrics Society and the Association of Directors of Geriatric Academic Programs. He served for 8 years on the American Board of Internal Medicine's Board of Directors, including as chair from 2010 to 2011. Since 2016, Dr. Reuben has served as a trustee of the American Board of Internal Medicine Foundation. In 2000, Dr. Reuben received the Dennis H. Jahnigen Memorial Award for outstanding contributions to education in the field of geriatrics and, in 2008, he received the Joseph T. Freeman Award from the Gerontological Society of America. He was part of the team that received the 2008 John M. Eisenberg Patient Safety and Quality Award for Research–Joint Commission and National Quality Forum, for Assessing Care of the Vulnerable Elderly. In 2012, he received the Henderson Award from the American Geriatrics Society. In 2012, Dr. Reuben received one of the first CMMI Innovations Challenge awards to develop a model program to provide comprehensive, coordinated care for patients with Alzheimer's disease and other dementias. In 2014, he was one of three principal investigators to be awarded a multicenter clinical trial (STRIDE) by the Patient-Centered Outcomes Research Institute (PCORI) and the National Institute on Aging (NIA) to reduce serious falls-related injuries; it is the largest grant that PCORI has awarded. In 2018, he was awarded a multisite

PCORI- and NIA-funded pragmatic trial to compare the effectiveness of health system–based dementia care versus community-based dementia care versus usual care. Dr. Reuben was cochair of the 2020 National Research Summit in Care, Services, and Supports for Persons with Dementia and their Caregivers. He is a member of the National Advisory Council on Aging for the National Institute on Aging. Dr. Reuben continues to provide primary care for frail older persons, including attending on inpatient and geriatric psychiatry units at UCLA, and making house calls.

Julie Robison, Ph.D., a gerontologist and health services researcher, is a professor of medicine and public health science in the Center on Aging at the University of Connecticut (UConn) School of Medicine. She conducts evidence-based health services research and intervention studies focused on aging families and long-term services, supports, and policy, using quantitative and qualitative research methods. Her research aims to improve quality of life and quality of care for people who need long-term services and supports (LTSS) and their families.

Dr. Robison is the director of the UConn Center on Aging's Evaluation and Population Assessment Core and Recruitment and Community Engagement Core. She studies how well LTSS funded by Medicaid, Medicare, and other public-sector sources affect health and well-being outcomes. Specific areas of expertise include effectiveness of LTSS for older adults and their families, designing evaluations of innovative LTSS designed to promote person-centered care and independent living, LTSS for individuals with dementia, and health disparities in the population needing LTSS. The results of her work have a direct impact on the implementation of policies and programs that serve extremely vulnerable populations in Connecticut and nationally.

Dr. Robison has served as principal investigator or coinvestigator on more than 60 funded research studies and regularly presents research findings in national and community forums. She has published more than 80 scientific articles and book chapters and many legislative and policy reports. Dr. Robison is the editor-in-chief of the *Journal of Applied Gerontology*, an international forum for research with clear and immediate applicability to the health, care, and quality of life of older adults, providing comprehensive coverage of all areas of gerontological practice and policy.

Eric Schneider, M.D., M.Sc., leads National Center for Quality Assurance's (NCQA's) measurement, research, and contracting agenda as executive vice president of the Quality Measurement and Research Group. In this role, he helps drive NCQA's efforts to create a more equitable health care system and to advance the move to digital quality measurement. Dr. Schneider came to NCQA from the Commonwealth Fund, where he was senior vice president for Policy and Research and a member of its executive management team. He has a long history with NCQA, most recently as cochair of its Committee on Performance Measurement. He served on that committee for more than 10 years, including 9 as cochair. Prior to his tenure at the Commonwealth Fund, Dr. Schneider was principal researcher at the RAND Corporation and held the RAND Distinguished Chair in Health Care Quality. As the first director of RAND's Boston office, Dr. Schneider built its highly regarded multidisciplinary team of health services researchers. As a professor at the T. H. Chan Harvard School of Public Health and Harvard Medical School, Dr. Schneider taught health policy and practiced primary care internal medicine for 25 years. Widely regarded as one of the nation's preeminent health services researchers, Dr. Schneider has authored more than 125 published, peer-reviewed research investigations and dozens of other scientific or medical research publications, reviews, chapters, editorials, and more. His work has focused on four aspects of health care quality: performance measurement methods; evaluation of quality and safety measurement in public reporting and financial incentive programs; use of health care quality measures to assess racial, ethnic, and socioeconomic disparities in health care quality; and evaluation of innovative approaches in health insurance, organization and financing of health care, and the organization of health care delivery. Dr. Schneider trained in health services research, public health, and primary care general internal medicine. He holds a bachelor of science, cum laude, in biology from Columbia University and a master of science from the University of California, Berkeley. He earned his medical degree from the University of California, San Francisco. He is a member of the AcademyHealth Board of Directors and a fellow of both the American College of Physicians and the National Academy of Social Insurance.

Meena Seshamani, M.D., Ph.D., is an accomplished, strategic leader with a deep understanding of health economics and a heartfelt commitment to outstanding patient care. Her diverse background as a health care executive, health economist, physician, and health policy expert has given her a unique perspective on how health policy affects the real lives of patients. She most recently served as vice president of Clinical Care Transformation at MedStar Health, where she conceptualized, designed, and implemented population health and value-based care initiatives and served on the senior leadership of the 10 hospital, 300+ outpatient care site health system. The care models and service lines under her leadership, including community health, geriatrics, and palliative care, have been nationally recognized by the Institute for Healthcare Improvement and others. She also cared for patients as an assistant professor of otolaryngology–head and neck surgery at the Georgetown University School of Medicine. Dr. Seshamani also brings decades of policy experience to her role, including recently serving on the leadership of the Biden–Harris Transition HHS Agency Review Team. Prior to MedStar Health, she was director of the Office of Health Reform at the U.S. Department of Health and Human Services, where she drove strategy and led implementation of the Affordable Care Act across the department, including coverage policy, delivery system reform, and public health policy. She received her B.A. with honors in business economics from Brown University, her M.D. from the University of Pennsylvania School of Medicine, and her Ph.D. in health economics from the University of Oxford, where she was a Marshall Scholar. She completed her residency training in otolaryngology–head and neck surgery at the Johns Hopkins University School of Medicine, and practiced as a head and neck surgeon at Kaiser Permanente in San Francisco.

Tisamarie Sherry, M.D., Ph.D., is a deputy assistant secretary in the Office of the Assistant Secretary for Planning and Evaluation (ASPE) at the U.S. Department of Health and Human Services (HHS). ASPE conducts policy research, coordinates policy across HHS, and advises the Secretary of HHS on policy development. Dr. Sherry leads ASPE's Office of Behavioral Health, Disability, and Aging Policy, which also coordinates dementia care research and policy across HHS through its role overseeing implementation of the National Alzheimer's Project Act, including convening the Advisory Council on Alzheimer's Research, Care, and Services, and updating the National Plan to Address Alzheimer's Disease. Her previous experience includes working as a policy researcher at the RAND Corporation, and as a primary care physician. Dr. Sherry is a health economist and general internist whose research has investigated health care delivery, financing, and policy strategies to improve the health and economic status of adults with chronic medical conditions. Dr. Sherry has also served as a fellow with the Centers for Disease Control and Prevention's Global AIDS Program, and has served on the National Academies of Sciences, Engineering, and Medicine's Committee on Identifying Disabling Medical Conditions Likely to Improve with Treatment. She received her B.A. in molecular biology and public policy from Princeton University, and her M.D. and Ph.D. in health policy (concentrating in economics) from Harvard University, and she completed residency training in internal medicine at Brigham and Women's Hospital.

Bruce C. Vladeck, Ph.D., currently serves as a senior advisor to the Greater New York Hospital Association and LiveOnNY, and he is a consultant to a number of other health care organizations. He is chairman emeritus of the Board of Medicare Rights Center and serves on the boards of Penn Medicine and the Mary Imogene Bassett Hospital. During his professional career, Vladeck held a number of senior positions, including assistant commissioner, New Jersey State Department of Health; president, United Hospital Fund;

administrator, Health Care Financing Administration (now called CMS); senior vice president, Mount Sinai Medical Center; and interim president, University of Medicine and Dentistry of New Jersey. At the Health Care Financing Administration, Vladeck was the principal federal official responsible for Medicare and Medicaid. Of his many accomplishments in that position, he is proudest of refocusing the organization on services to beneficiaries. Previously, Vladeck also served as full-time faculty at Columbia University and the Mount Sinai School of Medicine, and as a trustee or director of many organizations, including New York City Health and Hospitals Corporation, Ascension Health, the Hadassah Hospital, the Kaiser Family Foundation, Health Care for the Homeless, the Primary Care Development Corporation, and the March of Dimes. He is also an elected member of the National Academy of Medicine, the New York Academy of Medicine, and the National Academy of Social Insurance. Vladeck received his B.A., magna cum laude, from Harvard College, and an M.A. and Ph.D. in political science from the University of Michigan. He is the author of *Unloving Care: The Nursing Home Tragedy* (Basic Books, 1980), still considered the standard reference on nursing home policy in the United States, and of more than 100 articles in the professional literature.

BIOGRAPHICAL SKETCHES OF PLANNING COMMITTEE MEMBERS

Richard G. Frank, Ph.D. (Chair), is a senior fellow in economic studies and director of the USC–Brookings Schaeffer Initiative on Health Policy. He is the Margaret T. Morris Professor of Health Economics, Emeritus, in the Department of Health Care Policy at Harvard Medical School. From 2014 to 2016 he served as assistant secretary for planning and evaluation in the U.S. Department of Health and Human Services. His research is focused on the economics of mental health and substance abuse care, long-term care financing policy, health care competition, implementation of health reform, and disability policy. Dr. Frank served as an editor for the *Journal of Health Economics* from 2005 to 2014. Dr. Frank was awarded the Georgescu-Roegen Prize from the Southern Economic Association, the Carl A. Taube Award from the American Public Health Association, and the Distinguished Investigator Award from AcademyHealth. He was elected to the Institute of Medicine (National Academy of Medicine) in 1997. He is coauthor with Sherry Glied of the book *Better but Not Well* (Johns Hopkins University Press, 2006).

Elisabeth Belmont, J.D., serves as corporate counsel for MaineHealth, which is ranked among the nation's top 100 integrated health care delivery networks and has combined annual revenues of nearly $2 billion. She is responsible for a myriad of complex issues faced by an integrated delivery system on a daily basis and has a specialty concentration in health information and technology. Ms. Belmont has participated in a number of national initiatives where quality improvement, patient safety, and information technologies intersect including events sponsored by the HHS Office of the National Coordinator, HHS Office of the Inspector General, American Health Lawyers Association, American Society of Healthcare Risk Management, and American Association for the Advancement of Science. She serves as a member of the Division Committee of the Health and Medicine Division of the National Academies of Sciences, Engineering, and Medicine. She is a former member of the National Academies' Board on Health Care Services of the Health and Medicine Division, and participated as a member of the National Academies' Consensus Study Committees on Improving Diagnosis in Health Care and Systems Approaches to Improve Patient Care by Supporting Clinician Well-Being. Additionally, Ms. Belmont is a past president of the American Health Lawyers Association, former chair of the Association's Health Information & Technology Practice Group, and former chair of the Association's Quality in Action Task Force. She was also appointed cochair of the National Quality Forum's Health IT Patient Safety Measures Standing Committee. She previously served on the advisory boards of Bloomberg's *Health Law Reporter* and *Health Law & Business News*. Ms. Belmont coauthored agency guidance, *EHR Contracts Untangled: Selecting Wisely, Negotiating Terms and Understanding the Fine Print*, for the HHS Office of the National Coordinator. She is the recipient of numerous honors, including being named by *Modern Healthcare* as one of the 2007 Top 25 Most Powerful Women in Healthcare, being selected to receive the American Health Lawyers Association 2014 David J. Greenburg Service Award, and being named by the National Academies of Sciences, Engineering, and Medicine as a 2016 National Associate for outstanding contributions to the work of the National Academies.

Terry Fulmer, Ph.D., R.N., FAAN, is the president of the John A. Hartford Foundation in New York City, a foundation dedicated to improving the care of older adults. Established in 1929, the Foundation has a current endowment of more than $650 million. She serves as the chief strategist for the Foundation, and her vision for better care of older adults is catalyzing the Age-Friendly Health Systems social movement. She is an elected member of the National Academy of Medicine and recently served on the independent Coronavirus Commission for Safety and Quality in Nursing Homes established to advise the Centers for Medicare and Medicaid Services. She previously served as distinguished professor and dean of health sciences at Northeastern University. Prior, she served as the Erline Perkins McGriff Professor and Founding Dean of the New York University College of Nursing. She received her bachelor's degree from Skidmore College, her master's and doctoral degrees from Boston College, and her geriatric nurse practitioner post-master's certificate from NYU. She completed a Brookdale National Fellowship, and she is the first nurse to have served on the board of the American Geriatrics Society. She is also the first nurse to have served as president of the Gerontological Society of America, which awarded her the 2019 Donald P. Kent Award for exemplifying the highest standards for professional leadership in the field of aging.

Scott D. Halpern, M.D., Ph.D., is the John M. Eisenberg Professor of Medicine, Epidemiology, and Medical Ethics and Health Policy at the University of Pennsylvania, and a practicing critical care doctor. He is the founding director of the Palliative and Advanced Illness Research Center, which generates evidence to advance policies and practices with the goals of improving the lives of all people affected by serious illness and removing the barriers to health equity that commonly face seriously ill patients. He is also director of the NIA-funded Penn Roybal P30 Center on Palliative Care in Dementia. His research awards include AcademyHealth's Alice S. Hersh New Investigator Award, the Young Leader Award from the Robert Wood Johnson Foundation, the American Federation for Medical Research's Outstanding Investigator Award for the best scientist in any field under the age of 45, and the Association of Clinical and Translational Science's Distinguished Investigator Award. His mentoring awards include the John Hansen-Flaschen Award for Outstanding Mentorship and the Arthur K. Asbury Outstanding Faculty Mentor Award. He is an elected member of the American Society of Clinical Investigation and the Association of American Physicians, an elected fellow of the Hastings Center, and serves on the editorial boards of the *Annals of Internal Medicine* and the *American Journal of Bioethics*.

Sharon K. Inouye, M.D., M.P.H., is the director of the Aging Brain Center at the Hinda and Arthur Marcus Institute for Aging Research, Hebrew SeniorLife in Boston, Massachusetts. She holds the Milton and Shirley F. Levy Family Chair and is a professor of medicine at Harvard Medical School (Beth Israel Deaconess Medical Center). Her research focuses on delirium and functional decline in hospitalized older patients, resulting in more than 300 peer-reviewed original articles to date. Currently, she is the overall principal investigator of the Successful Aging after Elective Surgery (SAGES) study, an $11 million program project on delirium funded by the National Institute on Aging, as well as other active research projects. The purpose of the SAGES study is to examine the interface of delirium and dementia, whether delirium alters the course of dementia, and whether delirium leads to long-standing cognitive impairment and pathologic changes in the brain. Dr. Inouye is committed to improving the health and quality of life for older persons and their families. Dr. Inouye developed and validated the Confusion Assessment Method, the most widely used instrument for the identification of delirium. She conceptualized the multifactorial model for delirium, which focuses on identification of predisposing and precipitating factors for delirium. Her work involves translating theories of clinical investigation into practical applications that directly improve the quality of life for older adults. She developed the Hospital Elder Life Program (HELP), a multicomponent intervention strategy designed to prevent delirium by targeting six delirium risk factors. HELP was successful in reducing delirium by 40 percent and was published in a landmark study in the *New England Journal of Medicine*. This study was the first to show that a substantial proportion of delirium is preventable. Additionally, HELP has been shown to reduce falls, functional decline, and hospital costs, and to improve patient, family, and nursing satisfaction. The HELP program has been adopted by hundreds of hospitals worldwide.

Faith Mitchell, Ph.D., is an institute fellow at the Urban Institute, working with the Center on Nonprofits and Philanthropy and the Health Policy Center. She is also developing Urban's American Transformation project, which looks at the implications—and possibilities—of this country's racial and ethnic evolution. Over several decades, her career has bridged research, practice, and social and health policy. Previously, Mitchell was president and CEO of Grantmakers In Health, a Washington, D.C.–based national organization that advises, informs, and supports the work of health foundations and corporate giving programs. Before that, she held leadership positions at the National Academies (National Research Council and Institute of Medicine), U.S. Department of State, William and Flora Hewlett Foundation, and the San Francisco Foundation. Mitchell has a doctorate in medical anthropology from the University of California, Berkeley. She has written or edited numerous policy-related publications and is the author of *Hoodoo Medicine*, a groundbreaking study of Black folk medicine. She cochairs the advisory group for the John A. Hartford Foundation/Institute for Healthcare Improvement Age-Friendly Health Systems initiative; serves on the advisory committee of the National Collaborative for Health Equity, the editorial board of *Health Affairs*, and the boards of directors of Community Wealth Partners and the Jacob & Valeria Langeloth Foundation; and is a member of the Board on Health Care Services of the National Academies of Sciences, Engineering, and Medicine.

Julie Robison, Ph.D., a gerontologist and health services researcher, is a professor of medicine and public health science in the Center on Aging at the University of Connecticut (UConn) School of Medicine. She conducts evidence-based health services research and intervention studies focused on aging families and long-term services, supports, and policy, using quantitative and qualitative research methods. Her research aims to improve the quality of life and quality of care for people who need long-term services and supports (LTSS) and their families.

Dr. Robison is the director of the UConn Center on Aging's Evaluation and Population Assessment Core and Recruitment and Community Engagement Core. She studies how well LTSS funded by Medicaid, Medicare, and other public-sector sources affect health and well-being outcomes. Specific areas of expertise include effectiveness of LTSS for older adults and their families, designing evaluations of innovative LTSS designed to promote person-centered care and independent living, LTSS for individuals with dementia, and health disparities in the population needing LTSS. The results of her work have a direct impact on the implementation of policies and programs that serve extremely vulnerable populations in Connecticut and nationally.

Dr. Robison has served as principal investigator or coinvestigator on more than 60 funded research studies and regularly presents research findings in national and community forums. She has published over 80 scientific articles and book chapters and many legislative and policy reports. Dr. Robison is the editor-in-chief of the *Journal of Applied Gerontology*, an international forum for research with clear and immediate applicability to the health, care, and quality of life of older adults, providing comprehensive coverage of all areas of gerontological practice and policy.

Appendix E

Acronyms and Abbreviations

AARP	American Association of Retired Persons
ACL	Administration for Community Living
ACO	accountable care organization
ACOVE-3	Assessing Care of Vulnerable Elders 3
AD	Alzheimer's disease
ADC	Alzheimer's and Dementia Care Program
ADRD	Alzheimer's disease and related dementias
AI	Artificial Intelligence
APM	alternative payment mechanism
ASPE	Office of the Assistant Secretary for Planning and Evaluation
BOLD	Building Our Largest Dementia Infrastructure for Alzheimer's Act
BRICC	Benjamin Rose Institute on Aging Care Consultation
BSR	National Institute on Aging Division of Behavioral and Social Research
CBO	community-based organization
CDC	Centers for Disease Control and Prevention
CMMI	Center for Medicare and Medicaid Innovation
CMS	Centers for Medicare and Medicaid Services
COPE	Care of Persons with Dementia in their Environments
COVE	Care of Vulnerable Elders

COVID-19	Coronavirus Disease 2019
CPT	Current Procedural Terminology
ED	emergency department
EHR	electronic health record
EMS	emergency medical services
EMT	emergency medical technician
GCBH	Global Council on Brain Health
GED	geriatric emergency department
GME	graduate medical education
HABC	University of Indiana Healthy Aging Brain Center
HCBS	home- and community-based services
HEDIS	Healthcare Effectiveness Data and Information Set
HELP	Hospital Elder Life Program
HIE	health information exchange
HIT	health information technology
HRSA	Health Resources and Services Administration
ICOPE	Integrated Care for Older People
ICU	intensive care unit
IHI	Institute for Healthcare Improvement
IMCC	Integrated Memory Care Clinic
JAHF	John A. Hartford Foundation
LTC	long-term care
LTCI	long-term care insurance
LTSS	long-term services and supports
MCI	mild cognitive impairment
MedPAC	Medicare Payment Advisory Commission
MFP	Money Follows the Person
MIND	Maximizing Independence (Johns Hopkins)
MOST	medical orders for scope of treatment
NACA	National Advisory Council on Aging
NAPA	National Alzheimer's Project Act
NCQA	National Center for Quality Assurance
NIA	National Institute on Aging

NIH	National Institutes of Health
NPO	nothing by mouth
OAA	Older Americans Act
OT	occupational therapy/occupational therapist
PACE	Program of All-inclusive Care for the Elderly
PCP	primary care provider
PCPI	Physician Consortium for Performance Improvement
PT	physical therapy/physical therapist
PTAC	Physician-Focused Payment Model Technical Advisory Committee
REACH II	Resources for Enhancing Alzheimer's Caregiver Health II
RN	registered nurse
UN	United Nations
VA	Veterans Administration
VBID	Value-Based Insurance Design
WHO	World Health Organization